Life Swap

About the authors

Jo Hampson

Jo was born in Sri Lanka in 1956. She was educated at Malvern and went to Nevilles Cross College, Durham. Following six years teaching in west London, Jo joined the Metropolitan Police Service in 1985. During her 15 years service with the police she served with the Met and she was seconded to the New South Wales Police, Australia where she worked on a cultural change programme with the service following a two year Royal Commission into police corruption. Her last posting was as a Chief Superintendent with Thames Valley Police.

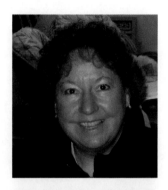

Georgina Perkins

Georgina was born in London in 1964. She was educated in Tunbridge Wells and after leaving school worked in the Magistrates Court Service until joining Thames Valley Police in 1987. Georgina was selected for Accelerated Promotion and when she left in 2001 she was working as a Detective Inspector.

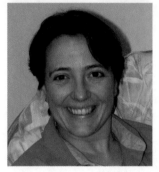

We would like to dedicate this book to Yvonne Bray - consultant psychologist, adviser and friend – with thanks for her expertise and enthusiasm for Stepping Off.

Our thanks to all the people who helped in the writing of this book, particularly those who allowed their stories to be used as case studies.

Simon and Wendy at Augill Castle, Brough, Cumbria
www.augillcastle.co.uk

Jane and Helen at La Maison Rose, Limousin, France
www.maisonrose.co.uk

Life Swap

The essential guide to downshifting

Life swap
ISBN 1 904601 43 X

First published in Great Britain in 2006 by Impact Publishing Ltd.
12 Pierrepont Street, Bath, BA1 1LA
info@impactpublishing.co.uk
www.impactpublishing.co.uk

A Cataloguing in Publication record for this title is available from the British Library.

Credits: Photo credits; Impact Publishing Ltd.

Printed in the UK by PIMS Print Crewkerne.

Foreword

In 2000, Jo Hampson and Georgina Perkins were fast-track senior Police Officers headed for the top of their profession. Then they gave it all up and downshifted to the country. Now they offer a unique service to others who want to do the same.

From their Cumbria retreat, at the top of Crosby Ravensworth Fell, Jo Hampson and Georgina Perkins ponder upon life as they gaze out on wonderful views overlooking the Lakeland Fells and the Pennines. In 2001, they gave up successful careers with the Police and bought a small business smoking food and making chocolates called The Old Smokehouse and Truffles. Following extraordinary success with this venture, they have drawn upon their skills and experience to launch 'Stepping Off' providing training and consultancy services for people wanting to change their lives for the better.

Jo started her working life as a primary school teacher in an inner city area. Five years later, she applied to join the Metropolitan Police. She soared rapidly to the rank of Chief Superintendent, having worked within National Police Training, the New South Wales Police in Australia and finally as Area Commander in Thames Valley where she was in charge of 400 staff and an annual budget of £12 million, with only 14 years service.

Georgina was an Inspector with only seven years service, working as an operational officer, Staff Officer to the Chief Constable and finally as Detective Inspector on the Major Crime Unit, investigating murders and armed robberies.

With a further 15 years service ahead of them and promotions anticipated, they decided to leave policing. They both enjoyed their work, but felt that there was more to life. Although they enjoyed their profession, neither wanted to continue in an environment where working 80 hours a week had become something to brag about.

They heard on the grapevine that a small artisan food-producing business was for sale near Penrith and so quite by chance in 2001, the two senior police officers found themselves smoking salmon, chicken and cheese!

Within three years they had increased the turnover 300%, built the business up into one of the best known smokehouses in the country, won 16 National Food Awards, gained clients like Fortnum and Mason and Harvey Nichols, and were smoking privately for members of the Royal family. As in all business, when you become successful, people want to buy you out and in 2004, they were made an offer they couldn't refuse! It was then the ideal opportunity to start 'Stepping Off', a life change consultancy geared to helping other people downshift or embark upon a life change.

Life Swap, puts all their experience and know-how about downshifting into one accessible guide.

CONTENTS

Chapter six: Reality check – the downside of downshifting

Chapter seven: Dream on – the upside of downshifting

Chapter eight: Ten top tips for a successful life swap

Chapter nine: Case studies

Introduction

What's wrong with modern life?

We have more money than ever before. We borrow more, at lower rates, to get the things we want now. There is endless technology to help us do things quicker. TVs give us the choice of 40 different programmes - some even let us watch more than one programme at the same time! We can fly to exotic places for the weekend for less than a train fare to the next town and talk to people 12,000 miles away as though they were in the next room. The list of advantages to modern life could go on, seemingly, forever. So why are we generally not happy? Why do we hear so much about families fleeing to live in another country or giving it all up for a different life?

The truth is, of course, that in our headlong rush to make more money, to fund more and better trips, cars, helpful gadgets, and lifestyle accessories, we have forgotten one thing. Time. We no longer have time for the things that arguably really do make us feel good like a meal with friends or family, spending time with children, relatives, friends and partners and outside interests such as reading, sport and other hobbies. Without time, money is increasingly unsatisfying.

What's wrong with your life?

Do you really have quality of life?

Do you lead a balanced life? Are you living or do you just exist? Are you controlled by your job and by the hours you work and feel that there is no time left for you? Is your life panning out as you wanted it to and is it giving you the rewards that you expected? Does your life satisfy you?

What does 'quality of life' mean to you?

Is your life satisfying you or do you feel that there is something missing? If you think about 'quality of life' does it represent the life you are living now? If leisure is important to you, do you have enough time and do you achieve what you want to in your leisure time? Or are there other things you wish you had time for? Do you have free time? Or are you cash/work rich and time poor?

Are there other things that you want to do?

Do you wish you had time to do other things, but feel that your life is dominated by work? Do you have an ambition that you are hoping to one day realise? Have you always wanted to work at doing something that is different from what you are doing now? Is your life on hold until you retire, when you have plans to do something completely different? Do you wish you had more control over what you do in your life and were able to do different things?

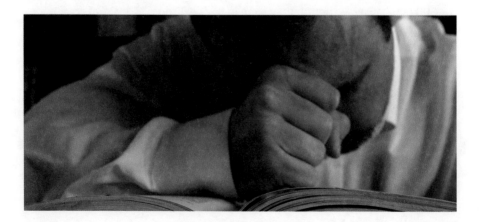

What is downshifting?

DOWNSHIFTING: *"Moving down a gear or changing to a simpler, less stressful life"*

Over the past decade, this expression has come to mean the move from a fast-track life to a more simple existence.

In 2002, 12% of 35 - 54 year olds were dreaming of trading a fast-paced job for a more balanced lifestyle; now people are actually doing it. Today, 4 out of 10 people under the age of 35 are planning to downshift from stressful jobs to a simpler life in the future.

Downshifting is becoming a very distinctive trend. There are tens of thousands of people who have already downshifted and many more who are planning to do so. In the UK, we are increasingly hearing about the migration of highly-skilled, hard-working people, often in very senior positions, who wish to leave the hard and fast, high-earning life in the Southeast or metropolitan conurbations for a more rural or even foreign destination to start living the 'good life'.

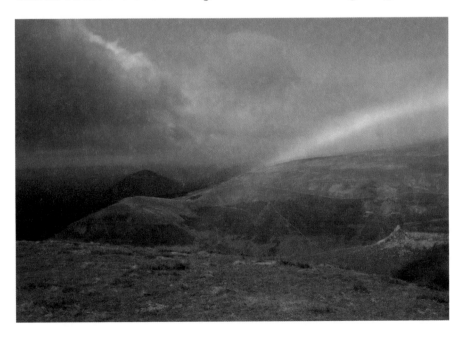

"Today four out of ten people under the age of 35 are planning to downshift from stressful jobs to a simpler life in the future."

The phenomenon of downshifting has been acknowledged for some time in the US. It has been widely recognised that in many instances, it is women who have been most likely to give up their busy careers and opt for a better quality of life. US research[1] has shown that there have been large numbers of women who were extremely successful, had broken through the glass ceilings and were about to achieve the highest positions in their chosen fields. These women, out of the blue, left their careers and dropped into 'oblivion'. It was thought that as these executives were becoming younger by the decade, they were leaving to start and bring up young families. However, this has proved to be incorrect. Instead, many of these women felt trapped and disenchanted with their careers and were fed up with compromising their own values. They were disillusioned about working for organisations who paid 'lip-service' to issues like equal opportunities and decided to downshift in an effort to regain control of their lives.[2]

In Australia, downshifting or voluntary simplicity as it is known there, is also a fast-growing trend. A number of academic studies suggest that a profound shift in values has impacted on the lives of ordinary Australians resulting in nearly 23% of working adults downshifting or simplifying their lives over the past decade. Here, people have chosen to live more simply on reduced incomes.

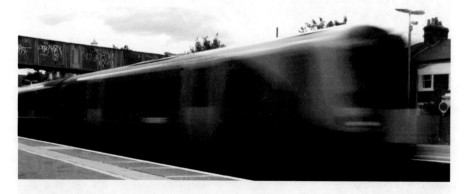

(1) Fortune and Yankelovich
(2) When work doesn't work any more - Elizabeth Perle McKenna

12

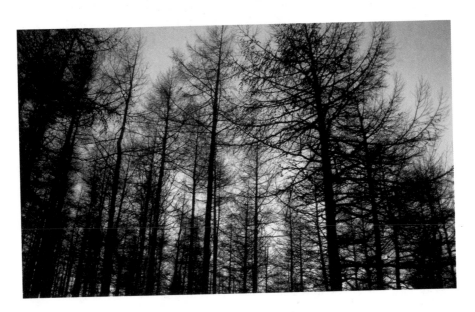

These people are not dropouts who have decided to quit mainstream society - it is a move right across the board, representing the full range of ages, incomes and social backgrounds.[3]

"Downshifters come from all walks of life".

Wherever downshifting is taking place, those making the move come from all walks of life. They may be people dissatisfied with their role, either in the public or private sector, approaching retirement, or facing redundancy. They may be looking to move from an urban area to a more rural one or they may just want a change and to enjoy life more. Many have ideas about going into business for themselves, or have specialist skills and talents which they want to use in their own creative environment.

Whatever the reason, people all over the western world are thinking about downshifting and swapping their lives for a more simple existence. Those who have actually made the life swap are reaping the benefits and are now enjoying a simpler, happier and better quality life.

(3) The Australian

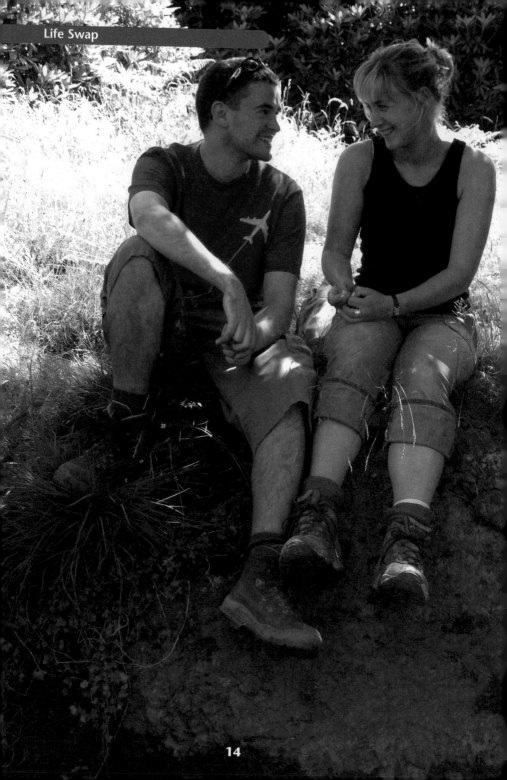

1

Do you really want to change your life?

How do you feel about your life now?

- Are you happy with your life?

- Is everything going well?

- Do you feel as though you have a balanced life?

- Do you have enough time to do the things you enjoy doing?

- Are you living the way you want to live?

- Do you feel that you are achieving everything that you set out to achieve?

- AND are you getting what you want out of life?

If your answer is yes to all these questions, then give this book to a friend instead!

If, however, the answer to some of the above questions is no or not really, or I'm not sure, then read on. Often people are fed up with the way their life is, but they are not sure why or how they came to be so fed up.

This book will help you discover why. Why you are thinking about swapping your life, what sort of life you would like to swap to and how to successfully achieve it. Follow the step-by-step activities in this book that will guide you towards a happier future.

Wake-Up Calls!

For whatever reason, we all seem to grow up with a work ethic which defines who we are as people. We fall into the trap of believing that we are defined by our work alone and that only by working hard and putting in long hours do we have any authority or worth. And then, we gather other commitments around us which make it impossible for us to change.

It is only when something dramatic happens that we may begin to question our lifestyle. Sadly, these moments are often tragic or devastating, like being nosed with a serious illness, being made redundant, having a heart attack or suffering the death of a family member or friend. We view these instances as a wake-up call. It is normally only when these things occur that we give ourselves permission to take a step back and really examine how we live our lives.

Give yourself permission to do what you want to do

It takes something dramatic to happen before we will give ourselves permission to question our quality of life. It takes even more thought and a degree of courage to allow ourselves permission to look outside of our lives to see if there could be another way to live, or a different way of living that will improve our quality of life.

The realisation that life is flying by and that we may not be making the most of it is a daunting thought.

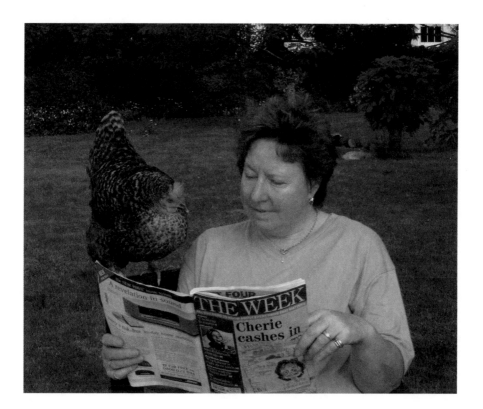

How do you feel about work?

Are you living to work or working to live?

Many of us now find ourselves working in a 'long hours' culture. The UK is slightly out of step with the rest of Europe in its working practices. How and why did we opt out of the '40 hour week' clause?

Do you work over 40 hours a week?

In many organisations, it is believed that working long hours will be rewarded. Those who put in the hours will get themselves noticed and will then have a better chance of promotion. The result is that we now have people boasting and bragging about the fact that they 'worked 75 or 80 hours last week'. For some, there is a mad rush to be seen to be the first in the office in the morning. Combine this with the reality that we are all working much harder than ever before. Everyone is striving to be a manager and organisations have streamlined their teams with the expectation that we will all do more. The outcome is that we have to be in the office by 7am to get the work done. It is inevitable that working in this sort of environment will cause high levels of stress.

Often, this culture is led and exacerbated by a few ambitious people at the top of the organisation.

"One senior executive that comes to mind used to have his clothes picked up by his driver at 5.30 am. He would then run the 5 kms into the office, shower and hold his first meeting over a 7.00 am breakfast at Simpson's in the Strand. All of which is fine if you have a driver, an office with a shower and enough income to pay for a restaurant breakfast everyday. However if you are working for this type of boss and are expected to be at that meeting, it is extremely stressful."

But it is also questionable whether this working culture is productive. It has been well researched and documented that we reach our peak in the morning and that we become increasingly less effective after we have been at work for longer than 8 hours. Productivity decreases and more mistakes are made when people work longer hours.[4] This research has obviously not reached the ears of some who sit round the boardroom table.

A recent survey found that more than one third of managers would cancel a holiday if something big at work came up and over half of these managers would cancel an anniversary dinner to work late if it was needed.[5]

1 hour a day less commuting reclaims 30 extra days a year!

Not only are we spending 10 - 12 hours a day at work, we are spending between 2 and 4 hours a day just getting there and back. How did we end up sitting in a traffic jam for 15 + hours every week? Never mind the stress of being held up, worrying about being late, trying to fill the time usefully by making phone calls or dictating notes into a machine; all of which increase the risk of driving into the car in front! If we are lucky we can commute to work by train. However having paid for the season ticket, for which you may have had to get a huge loan from the bank, the chances of getting a seat are almost non-existent, and you can't make yourself heard on your phone or dictaphone because everyone else around you is shouting into their phone or dictaphone!

It has to be accepted that the majority of our week will normally be spent at work, but that does not have to mean that work should dominate our lives or drag us down. Are we here just to spend our lives working or should work give us the means to live our lives?

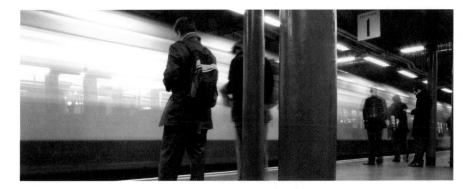

(4) Babbar and Aspelin 1998: Hirschman 2000: Shepard and Clifton 2000.
(5) Bibby Financial Services

How do you measure success?

Your life is fine - you are doing everything that is expected of you. You have a good job, you earn enough money, your family are doing well, you are happy in your house, you can afford a holiday, you like the car you drive and you are proud of what you have achieved. Well done - you have made it.

What is 'IT'?

The really big question for most people then is "What is 'IT'"? What does 'IT' feel like? Not many of us ever have the experience of being able to sit back and say, hand on heart - "Great - I've made it" and be completely satisfied with the result!

It is that awful realisation that you have done everything that has been asked of you, or that you have asked of yourself and yet, when you stop to take breath and look at what you have achieved, it just doesn't seem enough. It doesn't feel as though you have made it. It doesn't feel like you thought it was going to feel. What is this 'IT' you have been chasing all these years and is 'IT' worth it?

What does 'IT' stand for in your life?

- The big house - but you spend so little time in it that you are not sure whether it is worth the trouble and expense anymore

- Giving your children the best money could buy, but now you have reached the stage that you rarely see them and are missing watching them grow up

- Being promoted to Executive by the age of 45, but you no longer enjoy or are motivated by your job

- Owning that vintage sports car, but you only take it out of the garage three times a year

- Luxury holidays, but you spend most of the time on the phone to the office

- Being asked to be chair of governors for your old school, but you don't have time to attend the meetings.

I have achieved nearly everything I set out to achieve – why do I not feel good?

In reality 'IT' is going to be different things to different people and for some, this Holy Grail will always be elusive.

The reason for this is that many of us start out our working life with a particular destiny in mind, working to a particular set of standards and values. What we find, is that some twenty years down the line, we are in a completely different place than we thought we would be.

Reasons for dissatisfaction

Workplace disillusionment

You have always valued honesty and integrity. You treat people as you would like to be treated. You appoint and promote people on their merit. You offer respect to your staff and boss and work hard to earn their respect in return. One day you start to think about your organisation and you realise that it is not an honest place to work. It is very competitive and nepotistic. It is a cut-throat environment where you may be made redundant at any time and the staff are treated as an expendable commodity, not as useful individuals.

As a child you may have watched one or both of your parents give all to their job to the detriment of their family, or you may have experienced one of them being made redundant. So as a young person, you decided that you would not be dominated by work; that you would enjoy your life, put your partner first, make sure that you are always there for your children and that you would never work for the sort of organisation that your parents worked for. But, you get swept along with your life and job. You are offered a new job, so you move and then you are offered a different position. Some time later you move to a different department and suddenly, you find yourself living and working in an environment that is just like your parents organisations. You are now making people redundant, you hardly see your children or your partner and you are a long way from where you thought your plans and dreams would lead you. This realisation may remain a subconscious one, but it still has the ability to cause you stress.

21

Work/life balance

Expressions like 'being on the treadmill' and being 'stuck in the rat race' have come about through people's frustration at feeling that they are always at work and never have enough time for themselves. It is a feeling almost of desperation; they feel they are in a rut and cannot see a way out.

Life is busy. There is not a moment to spare and yet, they know that there are loads of other things they would rather be doing. A lot of people are waiting and planning for the day they retire, when they are going to do all those wonderful things they have always dreamed about. They feel as though life is on hold, they are treading water, waiting for the day when they can get off the treadmill and have some time for themselves.

Working towards someone else's goals

Sue's Story

Sue has been working as a secretary for a number of years. She hates it. She wanted to go to Drama College, but her career advisors and parents persuaded her to go to secretarial college first so that she would 'always have something to fall back on'. She did go to Drama College, but found it difficult to make a living, so she got a job as a highly-paid secretary. Much of her stress and unhappiness at work comes from the fact that at the back of her mind, she thinks she has failed because she has had to 'fall back on' her secretarial skills.

It is hard for a young person to have the courage of their convictions. Many people are brought up to think that their elders know what is best for them. Therefore, there is huge pressure to conform and comply. Sue eventually went to Drama College, but she went in the knowledge that it was disapproved of by those who held positions of authority in her life, and her failure to succeed almost confirmed in her own mind that they had been right. This created double the pressure and made it very difficult for her to get out and try something different.

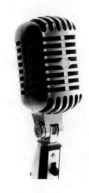

Bob's Story

Bob is working as an engineer because his father told him it would be a good grounding and that he would always get a job. Bob's father was a manual worker and wanted something better for him. He knew his son had the ability to achieve more in his life and he wanted to make sure that he had the opportunity. All Bob ever wanted to do was play music and have his own recording studio. Twenty years later, Bob has a top executive position, a high salary and a beautiful house, but is not happy at work because it was his father's choice and not his own.

Bob spent years living someone else's dream. He led the life his father had wanted to lead. He obeyed his father knowing that his family had sacrificed a lot for him to go through university. It was, therefore, hard for Bob to get out and start something different.

Both Sue and Bob were constrained by their family's definite outlook on life. They conformed to what their parents thought was best for them and they did it to please their families. This is very common. It is difficult for a young person to go against everything they have been brought up to believe, even if they feel differently inside. When we are young, we don't tend to have any perspective on our own qualities and we trust those who are around us. The result is that we lead an external life that is different to how we feel inside and in many instances we try to hide or bury who or what we want to be.

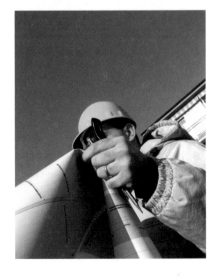

It is only when people reach a stage where they can give themselves permission to think about an alternative lifestyle that their early ambitions come to the fore. Partly spurred on by a desire to negate their regrets and also because of the shortened time left to achieve these or other ambitions, there is a huge release and they approach their life swap with enormous energy and exhilaration.

Not having control

Our lives today are complex and busy. We never seem to have enough time to fit in all that we want to do and we often find ourselves responding to things which are beyond our control. Most of us are dominated by our work. Understandably we work the hours the bosses need us to work, rather than the hours that suit us and we work extra hours, beyond those of our contract.

In a recent survey it was discovered that nearly five million UK workers work an average of 8 hours unpaid overtime a week! [6]

Many people, even in junior management positions stay late to finish work or take work home to finish in the evenings or at the weekends.

Being tied into your work beyond 9-5, Monday – Friday, can be a cause of stress. There are few jobs that allow you to go to work at nine o'clock and finish at five o'clock, leaving all thoughts of work behind you. While some people love being 'married' to their job and live to work, most people would prefer to work to live and be able to balance the time they spend at work and home better.

Of course, we would all say that we have complete control over our lives, but when you have a stressful job, your life often isn't your own. How guilty do you feel if there is some minor crisis at home and you have to leave an important meeting to sort it out? If you put yourself first, you can sometimes be seen as letting the side down or not having your priorities right. What impression will that give your boss if you are ambitious for promotion?

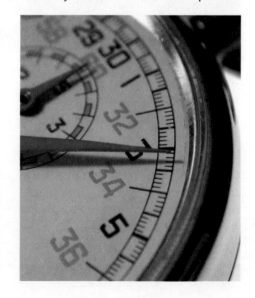

There is an automatic assumption that your work and the company or organisation should always come first. You are governed by your job and everything else has to come second. Something else has control over you!

(6) TUC

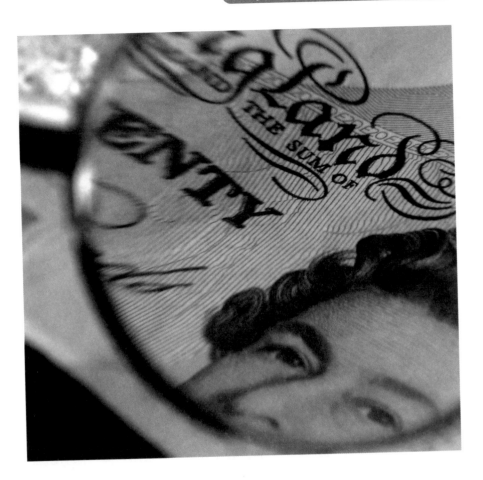

Money

To most of us, money is a significant factor in our working life, but it can become over-important. Surprisingly, there are an increasing number of people for whom money just does not do 'IT' any more. In fact, having the lifestyle that their money buys them is what is making them disillusioned and increasing their stress levels. This may sound strange, but subconsciously some people know that despite the fact that their money buys them all the material things that they want, it is not giving them other things that are equally if not more important. Things that money cannot buy – time, control over how they work, health, happiness, spiritual and intellectual fulfillment and more.

Jo's Story

Jo talks animatedly about going out for dinner. She said that she worked such long hours that it was normally about 9pm before she got home. Often she hadn't had time to go shopping or had forgotten to take something out of the freezer, so she and her partner just went to a nearby restaurant for dinner. It was an automatic thing to do. Hungry - no food - go to the nearest restaurant - satisfy hunger - cost was not an issue. However, one day she remembered what it used to feel like to go out for a meal. How, when she was living on a meagre wage, going out for dinner was a real treat, something to look forward to, to get dressed up for, to be savoured and enjoyed.

She had lost that feeling completely and she began to resent the fact that by having money and the lifestyle to go with it, she was no longer able to enjoy some of the 'simpler' things in life.

Going out for a meal is just one example of something that used to be a treat, but was now just part of the rushed daily routine. Jo found that her value systems were changing. Over the years, she had moved away from what really mattered to her. She realised that the way she was now living did not guarantee enjoyment and fulfillment in her life. She had been swept away on the crest of a materialistic wave and deep down she knew she was living a hollow life and achieving little that really meant anything to her. Having money had not brought her all that she longed for, it was not all wonderful and pleasurable, it just allowed her to survive better day-to-day in a job that she didn't enjoy anymore.

These are some really complex issues about why we may be successful in our working lives and yet continue to be disillusioned and disenchanted with our lot.

It is important to try and find out why you are disillusioned with your working life. If you don't know what it is you are unhappy with, you may find yourself jumping out of the frying pan and into the fire when you finally do change your life.

2

Why do you want to change your life?

We have come to think that downshifting is normally about leaving the job in the city and moving to a rural location; about buying a smallholding, growing vegetables and keeping chickens. Actually, downshifting is broader than that; people downshift for a multitude of different reasons and to do a multitude of different things.

There are of course lots of reasons why people look at changing their lives and not all of them are about work. Maybe, you have found that you and your partner no longer live together; you just cohabit. You spend your lives ferrying the kids around, walking the dog, fetching groceries, decorating the house and maintaining the garden, so that by the time you do sit down in the evening you have absolutely no energy to focus on anything other than the television. You are dreading going back to work and are disappointed that all you have done are the chores. You have not had any time for fun or to do the things you want to do. For you, it is about finding a way to manage all the different things that you need to do at home and find the discipline to factor in some time for you and/or your partner and the other things you enjoy.

No two people downshift for exactly the same reasons, but here (opposite) are ten of the most common reasons which push people to change their lives.

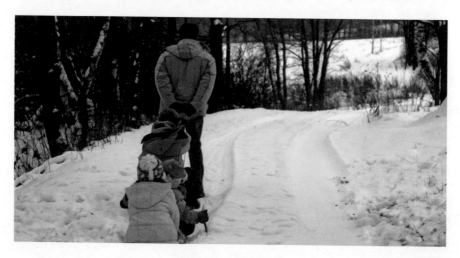

10 reasons why people want to downshift

1   They feel that their work/life balance is wrong – their life is dominated by the hours they work and they don't feel that they have enough time for other things. They are fed up with living to work when they want to work to live

2   They feel they do not have control of their life – their life is not their own and they are controlled by the demands of others

3   They are facing redundancy – they suddenly have no job security and realise that their fate is in someone else's hands. This is an opportunity to do something they have always wanted to do

4   They want to fulfill their potential – they have long had an ambition to do something different and they feel that time is running out

5   They are fed up with city living - with the hustle, bustle and pace of the crowded city

6   They want to start their own business – they have an ambition to set up on their own and work for themselves

7   They want to move to the country or abroad – they feel as though they want to get away and live a completely different life in a completely different place

8   They feel life is passing them by – something happens to make people think about their life, their work and their need to achieve something before it is too late

9   They just want to live a simpler life – they are fed up with the pressure and stress of living a modern complex life and they want to give their family a chance to live a simpler, quieter and less complicated existence

10 They are fed up with the rat race – with a life that feels as though they are on a roller coaster that they cannot get off. They cannot see a light at the end of the tunnel.

So, we can see that the motivating factors to make a life change are numerous.

Have a look at this questionnaire and see where you score in our downshifting range.

	Yes	No
Do you feel you are not always in control of your life?		
Do you resent the time spent commuting to work?		
Have you ever thought about working for yourself?		
Do you dream of living a different life?		
Do you ever wish that you might be offered redundancy?		
Do you ever think you would like to settle in a more rural or different area?		
Do you feel set apart from some of your colleagues?		
Are you unhappy with your work/life balance?		
Have you ever discussed the option of doing something different with a partner or friend?		
Do you work late in the evenings or at weekends?		

	Yes	No
Do you have to bring work home?		
Have you ever dreamed of living the 'good life'?		
Do you ever think that your values may be different to that of your colleagues or the organisation?		
Do you wish you had more leisure time?		
Do you think about starting a new career?		
Is there something you really want to do, but you are putting it off until you retire?		
Have you had to cancel a social arrangement to go to work in the past six months?		
Do you dream about having a simpler life, even if it means earning less?		
Are you dissatisfied with your quality of life?		

Does work affect who you are?

A key issue, which is being addressed in this questionnaire, is – 'how satisfied are you in your life?' Do you feel that your work dominates your life? Do you feel 'in hock' to your organisation? Do you feel as though your work owns you? Does your work allow you to be you and have your own life and priorities or do you suppress your real personality and interests, in order to be seen to fit in and get on? Are you a different person at home to the one who goes to work?

Now, check out your score below -

You are happy where you are

0 -5 – If you answered YES between 0-5 times then you are probably like most of us, a bit disgruntled with work but essentially happy with life. You are able to cope with the highs and lows at work and maintain a reasonably happy balance at home.

You are sitting on the fence

5 -10 – If you answered YES between 5-10 questions then you are more than normally 'fed up with work'. You are on the verge of considering a new lifestyle, but somehow you don't feel that things are quite bad enough to make the move.

You are teetering on the edge

10 -15 – If you answered YES between 10-15 then there is some serious dreaming going on and you certainly need to give yourself permission to think that a life-swap might be a real possibility.

Ready to take the leap!

15 + – If you answered YES to more than 15 then you are a serious contender for improving your quality of life and living in a different way.

Steps to help you make that life-changing decision.

The real point of the test is, of course, not just how many you answered yes to, but more importantly, it's about WHICH ones you answered yes to.

Step One: What frustrates you?

This step will help you look at your life; particularly your working life. By looking at your answers to the questionnaire, you will begin to pinpoint exactly which areas are causing your frustration.

Activity

Have a look at your answers. Write down the list of all the questions you answered yes to. What do you see? Is there a pattern? They will help pinpoint the reasons why you want to change your direction.

If you answered yes to the questions about working for yourself or doing something different, you may be looking to branch out on your own.

However, if you answered yes to the questions about wanting more spare time, or resenting the time spent commuting to work, then it may be that what is behind your discontent are the time demands your job places on you and therefore, you should look at your work/life balance, your time management and possibly your job location.

If you can find a common thread in your answers it will go some way to helping you understand what the specific things are that are making you want to get out and change your life.

Important Hint

You don't have to downshift completely to improve your life. There are many ways in which you can start to live differently which could give you a real sense of satisfaction, freedom and achievement.

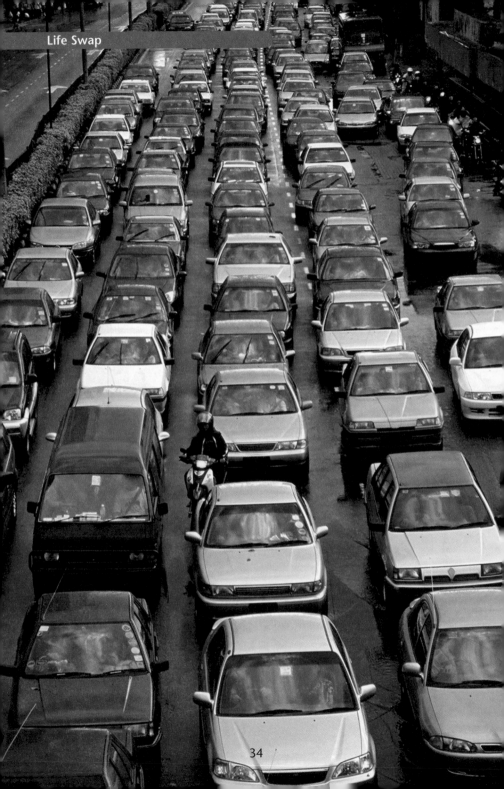

3

Discover what is making you dissatisfied with life

Life-changing moments

Life-changing moments are different from the wake-up calls. These are small events that happen in your life to which you have an abnormal reaction. These moments can be any number of things from being criticised at work, missing an important event because of a traffic jam or a comment made by someone either at work or home, to watching an exceptional film or reading an inspiring book. It is the moment, when in a flash you see your life from a different perspective and you suddenly ask yourself the question "what am I doing?"

Life-changing moments are when something happens that makes you suddenly realise that your life is not turning out as you planned. Here are just a few of the most common reactions.

- You look at what is happening around you and for the first time really think 'this is not for me anymore'
- You realise that you are no longer completely in control of the different demands on your life
- You feel that you don't want to put up with all the stress and anguish anymore
- You suddenly feel really angry within; you say 'to hell with it, I want out'.

These moments are a revelation. Was it the moment of utter disappointment when you made it to your son's sports day, but actually missed his race because you were on your mobile to the office? Perhaps it was finding out about a friend's illness, or realising that you were being undermined at work, or learning that what you believed were the good points about your job are slowly being eroded. Maybe you are just tired of the same old day-to-day drudgery. In many cases, it is about that ultimate realisation that you have no control over your life and its direction. You ask yourself the question, if it all ended now would I be happy with what my life has been?

Usually, we manage to get over these moments and once the stress levels have dropped again or the anger has passed, we begin to relax back into the normal chaos, happy to have survived and be back in our comfort zone.

For some people, however, these life-changing moments begin a sub-conscious reaction. The thoughts start escalating, and 'I want out' starts to turn into 'not only do I want out, but I can get out'! They realise that they only have one shot at life and they need to regain control of their future.

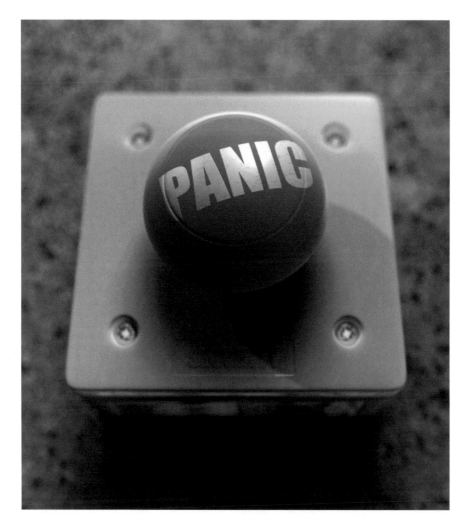

Do any of these sound familiar?

Lack of support and encouragement

Graham

Graham, who worked in public service, was recently promoted to a new senior position where he was in charge of five departments. He was tackling an almost vertical learning curve, working long hours, thoroughly enjoying it and earning a good wage. He relished the challenge of managing a large number of staff and he cared about being a good manager and supporting individuals. He was well-respected by his staff and was doing well.

He was one of a team of eight managers all on the same grade. He arranged to meet with his boss in the first week. He was expecting to talk about his new position, what was going to be expected of him and the direction his boss wanted him to take his section of the organisation. As it turned out, his boss was too busy to meet him, so he relied on his other team members for any assistance he needed. However, the level of competition between these people was such that he found very little assistance forthcoming and there was even less support.

Graham was asked to represent the organisation at a meeting with some important potential clients and show them what work his section undertook. Graham was shocked that he had been picked as he was the new kid on the block and he felt that this was an unnecessary burden on him and his department. However, he accepted and began to plan the meeting.

He tried several times to meet with his boss, to sound out ideas and gain advice, but his boss was always too busy. The only time his boss made contact with him was in the middle of the meeting with the clients, interrupting Graham's presentation with a phone call. The purpose of the call was to demand to know why Graham's department hadn't hit their performance targets that week!

Graham was good at his job and was destined for the top of his profession, but that phone call was a life-changing moment for him. He felt totally isolated, unsupported and let down. He knew that as an executive he had moved into the 'big boys league' but he never believed that the organisation, which sold itself

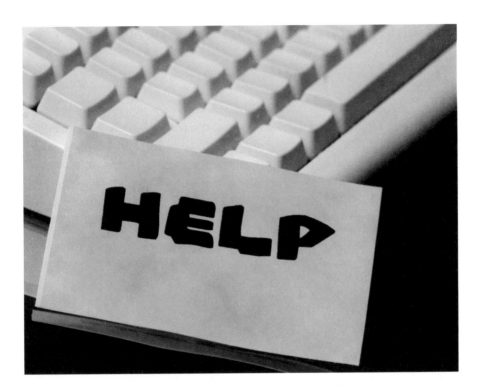

as a caring one, would treat people in such a way. Now Graham may have been slightly naïve, but that phone call started him thinking about the possibility of getting out and starting again, of leading a different life.

Graham was successful and good at his job. He worked hard and supported and respected his colleagues and the organisation. What he expected was a level of support and respect in return. When he needed and looked for it, it wasn't there. He felt isolated and abandoned. He was criticised if he did something wrong, but was never praised or encouraged when he did something right. When he wanted and needed advice, his managers were too busy to help him.

This increased Graham's stress levels. He became disillusioned with the organisation. He was disappointed that what he had been taught about looking after and supporting staff was not shared by others in the organisation. He lost respect for his bosses and found he no longer wanted to work in that sort of environment.

Working towards someone else's goals

Gillian

Gillian was a busy working Mum. She worked for a small company doing admin and accounts. When she started, all she really wanted was a comfortable job, working 9-5 where she didn't have to bring work home or worry too much about the office – after all her family was the most important thing in her life. As the company grew, so did Gillian's job. She was often still in the office past 6pm, she had taken on extra work to help the company plan an expansion, and she brought work home in the evenings.

Gillian rather liked this extra responsibility and she had been promised a small bonus at the year-end. But she found her stress levels increasing for the first time in her working life and managing her work and children was becoming difficult. She felt she was being pulled in several different directions at once and she was conscious that her husband was beginning to resent the time she spent on work in the evenings and at the weekend.

One evening, she was sitting in the kitchen at about 9pm finishing off some paperwork as her husband was out that evening. It had been a really hectic day.

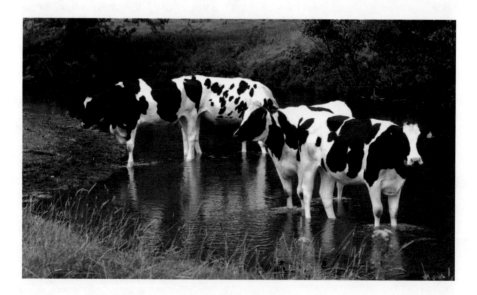

She had almost forgotten that it was the kids' night at Scouts, so she had rushed to pick them up and take them home. She then immediately sat down and got on with her work. Her son came in and started bothering her. She was annoyed and told him to stop messing about and go to bed. 'Bed?' he said looking taken aback. 'We can't go to bed yet we haven't had any supper'.

Not surprisingly this was a life-changing moment for Gillian. She had become so wrapped up in the demands of work that the very things she had always said were most important to her were being neglected.

UK workers contribute £23 billion of unpaid overtime to their work. [7]

Gillian had got her work/ life balance wrong. She had started out with a clear definition that her job was just a job and that her life outside work was more important. Her life-changing moment made her realise that her job had taken over. She was working towards someone else's goals. Her marriage, children and social life were suffering and all she was doing was working. She was no longer living her life in the way she wanted to live it. Subconsciously, she had been aware of this and this may have been causing her stress, but it was the occasion of her children's supper that allowed this thought to become a conscious and obvious one.

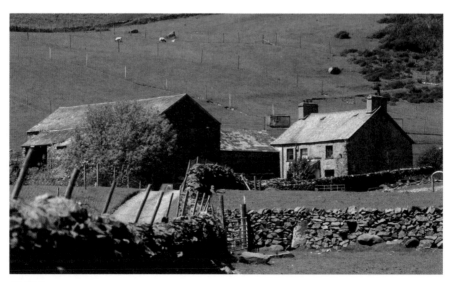

(7) TUC

Loss of faith in the organisation

Robin

In 1993, Robin was working as a supervisor in a large organisation. One day, one of the women working for him put in a complaint about the behaviour of another member of the team. Robin tried to support the complainant with very little assistance from senior management who were more concerned with limiting 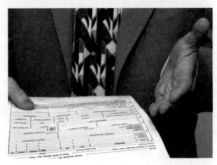 the damage to the organisation. He did what he could, but felt that there was a lack of awareness about these situations and that as a result the complainant had become more distressed. Eventually, through an internal process, the matter was concluded. Robin felt that the organisation would benefit from learning from the experience and he wrote a report setting out some simple guidelines about how to deal with such situations. The senior executives claimed to welcome his report and he was told that they would implement his recommendations as policy.

In 2000, Robin was again in a similar situation. Again he tried to support a complainant. He found the same issues re-occurred and in spite of his report seven years earlier, and repeated follow-ups, no official policy had ever been put in place and the organisation made as many mistakes this time as it had in 1993. For Robin, finding out that nothing had changed was a life-changing moment. He felt that his efforts had all been in vain.

In Robin's story we see someone who cares about his colleagues. He also cares about the organisation he works for. When he has the opportunity to do something good and worthwhile, he does it. He is praised for his initiative. However, the realisation that the management team had only paid lip service to his ideas, caused him to lose faith in the organisation. He no longer trusted the people he worked for. This lack of trust subtly alienated him from his colleagues and damaged his future with the organisation.

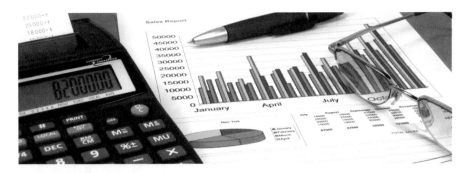

Living with the wrong work/life balance

Anna

Anna worked as a sales manager running a large team. She had booked to go away on holiday. The night before she went away she was still in the office at 11pm finishing off her work. She caught her flight the next day. Anna did very little for the first three days other than sleep. Throughout the rest of her holiday she received phone calls from her boss about issues back in the office. She was faxed a number of papers to read for a meeting to be held the day she returned and when she got back, she had to work an 80 hour week just to catch up.

Anna vowed never again to take a two-week holiday, as being away from her office caused her too much stress and extra work. The whole experience was a life-changing moment for Anna.

60% of managers fail to take their full holiday entitlement. [8]

Anna was simply working too hard and not giving herself time for leisure activities or friends and family. Her work/life balance was wrong and she was consumed with work. Her organisation dominated her personally and work dominated her life.

68% of people respond to their boss's requests whilst on holiday and 43% of people checked their work emails. [9]

(8) TUC
(9) ibid

43

Compromising your values

Margaret

Margaret was working in a large retail organisation. She didn't earn very much, but it got her out of the house now that her children had grown up and she enjoyed it. One day, her manager called all her team together and told them that because of new legislation they were going to have to change the way they worked. They were given a pack to read to learn all about the new system changes.

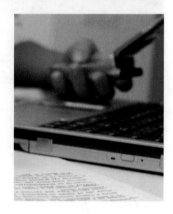

Margaret took all the new information home and read it. When the day came, she understood how things were going to alter and was ready for the changes. However, her supervisor obviously hadn't bothered to read up on the new legislation and didn't have a clue about how to implement the changes.

There was chaos. Margaret ended up doing the supervisor's job and helping everyone else implement the new systems. This was a life-changing moment for Margaret. She realised that, although she didn't have a very important job, she did care about and take her work seriously and wanted to do her best. Most of the people around her didn't seem to care about getting things right, about the standard of their work or about whether the organisation complied with the law or not. She realised at that moment that what she believed in was at odds with her workplace and fellow workers. She had far more ability than she had perhaps thought and her loyalty and commitment were not recognised in the environment where she worked.

Some people might say that Margaret had an old-fashioned work ethic. She was honest, reliable and did her job to the best of her ability. However, the system changes at work made her feel rather out on a limb. Suddenly, her set of values seemed out of synch with her fellow-workers. She stood up for what she believed in, but her work was compromised by those around her who had a different set of values. She had also perhaps under-estimated her own worth.

Competition

Peter

Peter had been headhunted to become Deputy Director of his department. It was a good job and he knew that he was being groomed to take over the Director's job when he retired. He was young, energetic, ambitious and highly thought of.

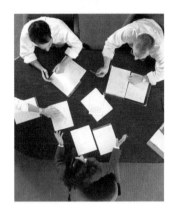

After about eight months in the role, there was a decision to amalgamate Peter's department with another department. Peter was not totally in favour of the idea as he felt that quality issues arose and that customer service might be compromised. However, the writing was on the wall and Peter got on with preparing his staff and department for the amalgamation. The question of who would be the Director of the new department was discussed and it was decided by the board that they would advertise the position. Peter applied. He felt confident as he had experience in both departments, while the Director of the other department was new to the organisation with little experience, having come from a completely different background.

Peter did not get the job and was made redundant. This was not a subtle life-changing moment. This was a huge shock that rocked Peter's world, but it enabled him to think about his life afresh, his job and the opportunity of living his future life in a different way.

Peter's story is simply one of competition. His story is by no means unique. Many people will identify with how Peter felt when he was made redundant. His situation is one of the most common reasons why people walk away from high-powered jobs and simplify their lives. Not all of them are actually made redundant but changes in work practices cause much the same damage.

How work can leave you feeling let down

These stories show a few of the different ways in which a life-changing moment can leave people feeling let down with their working life. On a subjective level, it is easy to empathise with these examples even though you may not have had the exact same experience.

The more fed up you become with your work, the more life-changing moments you will experience and the more frequent these life-changing moments will occur.

What happens when organisations move the goal posts

How many people do you know who work hard and do everything that is asked of them? Peter did. He completed all the training and got all the experience that he needed for promotion and then the organisation changed the rules.

Generally one of two things will happen:

Either

The organisation moves the goal posts for promotion. So today, if you had created X amount of sales, or gained X amount of experience or qualifications you would be almost guaranteed the next level or scale. Suddenly, there is a new head of HR and tomorrow promotion only comes through an assessment centre which does not take into account everything you have been working towards like experience or qualifications. You are now competing on a different playing field.

Or

They start giving the higher paid jobs to people who may be 10 years younger than you or who are from outside the industry. Suddenly, all your work and years of experience stand for nothing and the new kids on the block are getting the spoils. The organisation has changed. What they value in their staff has changed and you are no longer competing on a level playing field.

Step two: Life-changing moments

Having read this chapter, the next step is to identify what your life-changing moments have been. These will help you understand in more specific terms what is the root cause of your frustrations and unhappiness. Once you have identified these, you will be more certain about what you don't want to take with you into your new life.

Activity

Spend time thinking about any life-changing moments you may have had over the past 12 months. The moment when you lost your temper at work, when you felt you were wrongly criticised or when you skipped an important meeting because you had just had enough.

Write them down

Think about what these moments felt like. Why did they affect you so badly? What was it about the situation that made you so angry, sad or disappointed?

It is only by analysing what caused these incidents and why you reacted so strongly to them that you can then begin to work out what is causing your frustration and unhappiness. Answer this and you will be closer to knowing what it is that is making you want to start again.

Only when you have begun to understand what creates your internal stress and tension, can you begin to think seriously about why and how you might change and achieve greater satisfaction from your future life. Identifying the things that cause your life-changing moments will help you identify what is bad in your life and what you need to leave behind when you move into your new life.

Important Hint

You need to know and understand where you have been before you can know where you are going.

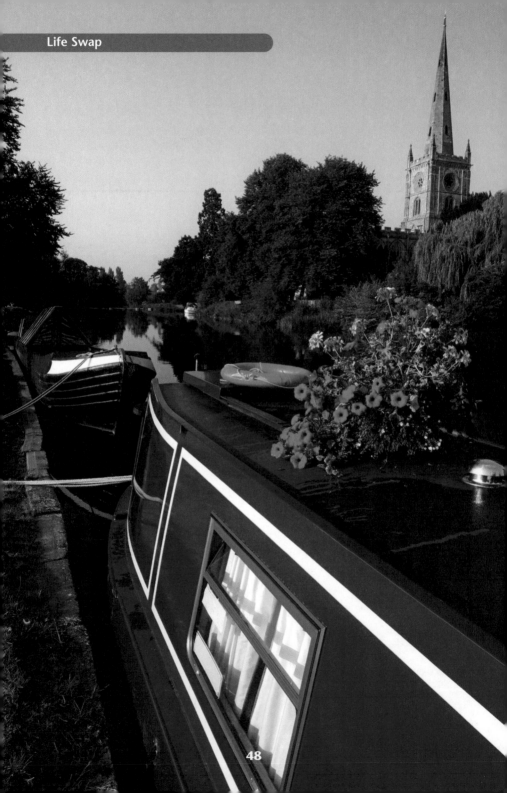

4

What life will you swap to?

What sort of downshifter are you?

Let's go back to the definition of Downshifting:

***"To move down a gear, or change to a simpler,
less stressful life"***.

There are two approaches to downshifting. You can either take your foot off the accelerator and slow down immediately as you would in an automatic car; or you can downshift in stages, slowing down to a different gear or down through the gears as you might in a manual car.

There are many degrees of downshifting and the route you take will depend on what sort of person you are. If you are a cautious driver, you might just downshift from fourth to third gear. This might mean that you keep the same job, but you make the decision never to bring work home. You might move out of the city, but be within commuting distance for work.

Some people, however, will just simply go for broke, give up their job, sell their house and move to a new life.

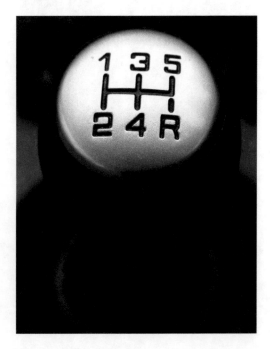

The analogy of the car and the gear system allows us to really look at the different ways we could downshift. Imagine life as a car journey. We are driving along, living our life, but then we become bored with the journey or something dramatic happens and we decide on a change of pace and direction. The issue now is how we approach the gear change and what gear we change to.

What kind of driver are you?

The Automatic downshifters

In downshifting terms, the drivers driving an automatic car will have come a long way down the road of thinking about what is causing angst and discontent in their lives. They will have been considering a life-change in one form or another for a long time - probably for longer than they actually realise.

Either – They will have spent a number of years dreaming about doing something different with their lives. We all know these people. They are the ones that have been coming up with hair-brained ideas about their future and different ways of making money (each idea is going to make them millions!); and they will probably have driven their families and colleagues mad with each new idea!

Or – These drivers have been increasingly fed up with their lot, but although they have been dreaming about giving it all up and starting again, they never actually believed that they could (or would) do it. In both of these instances, something will happen, they will have a life-changing moment, and both of these sets of people will just do it. The foot comes off the accelerator and the car will stop very quickly.

They are likely to come up with an idea, give in their notice, put it into practice and go for it, all in a very short space of time. They downshift in a dramatic way, up sticks and move, take a huge drop in salary, occasionally start up on their own or drop out completely to restore an old house.

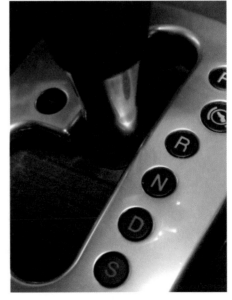

Maybe they are looking for the good life or the freedom that going it alone or working for themselves can provide. They find a way of life that matches their beliefs.

The Manual downshifters

Now what happens to those people who drive the manual car? They will be a little more cautious when thinking about what is causing angst and discontent in their lives. But they will have been considering a life-change in one form or another.

These people will downshift in a different way. They may not go the whole hog and come to a complete standstill. They may work their way down through the gears; just slowing down in incremental stages until they are in a more comfortable position.

What gear are you living in – and what gear would you like to be living in?

Most importantly, it does not matter which gear you live in as long as you know why you are in that gear and what it is about that gear that satisfies your needs and makes you happy. Embarking on a life swap begins with the realisation that you are not happy with your pace of life.

There are no right or wrong answers; people have to be happy in their own skin. There are no judgements being made in this book. If you are motivated by money then that is fine. Working hard and playing hard is a compromise you accept, enjoy and thrive on. The problem comes when you are living a life which doesn't prioritise what is important to you; when you are living a fast-paced life and working long hours to support a lifestyle which you never wanted in the first place.

Fifth gear

 People in this gear are racing through life in overdrive. They could be on cruise control, but it is fast and on track. They may be zipping through chicanes and accelerating through sharp bends. They are definitely living in the fast lane.

This requires immense concentration, commitment and dedication. It is unwise to take your eye off the road. In fact, it takes nearly all of your time just to keep going.

People who live in this gear are fuelled by work, possessions, fast cars, expensive food, the big house and exotic holidays. Generally, money, status, power and possessions are their motivation.

Great for some, but after a while others just get tired and not changing down the gears to accommodate the bends and road conditions can cause serious problems.

Fourth gear

Acknowledging that the fast track is just not for them anymore is, for many, the biggest step they will ever take. They still want the job, the money and the lifestyle, but they also want to work a little less and enjoy life a little more. So they make the decision to slow down a little, take a slightly less high-powered job, earn a little less money or just simply start to live their life differently.

They improve their time management and start to work smarter not harder. They spend time working out what their real priorities are and then they dedicate more time to those priorities and a little less time to work.

These people enjoy the good things in life. They are successful in material terms and enjoy the quality of the things around them. But they are becoming increasingly aware of the impact that their lifestyle is having on themselves, society and the environment. After a while, they may feel the need to ask themselves some searching questions and as a result may wish to slow down a bit and move away further from their present life.

These people don't want to downshift, but they do want to slow down a little and live a bit differently.

Third gear

Third gear people come in many guises. They could be those people who have always lived in third gear. They may have looked at the fast lane and thought that this is not for me. Alternatively, they may have been in the fast lane and then made the decision to move down a couple of gears in an effort to simplify their lives.

They may not have left their job, but they are not in the fast lane and they will definitely be managing their time better to include more leisure time. They could be inspired by the concept of 'green living'. They may not have moved house, but they will have started to live in their home differently. One of the cars may have gone from the garage and been replaced by two mountain bikes. Or the garage itself has gone and in its place there is a workshop or studio. Some of the garden may have been given over to a small vegetable patch, which is next to a large composting bin, and there may be solar panels on the shed roof.

This gear may be the most comfortable for the largest percentage of people, but it is also, possibly, the hardest to achieve. It is a real challenge to maintain a standard of living which also allows you to live simply and at your own pace. In this gear, there is a feeling of having regained some control of life and an acknowledgment that time is being spent doing what is important to them.

These people like their security. Generally they are not risk takers. They do want to change, but they don't want to lose too much. They are optimistic and believe that they can actually have it all. By working smarter they find they can achieve a purer lifestyle and a good standard of living by doing what they believe in. For those who have moved down to this gear, it is a happy medium. They have made a significant change in their lives, but not so significant that they are living completely differently.

Second gear

This is now becoming a seriously simple life. The fast track has been left far behind. The smart job and house have gone and the contents of the house have been squeezed into a smaller, more sensible residence in a quieter location. The air is cleaner, the schools are smaller, the salaries are much smaller, but then so are the outgoings.

There is room in the garden for a big vegetable patch - in fact the vegetable patch takes up most of the garden. In the corner where there are no vegetables, there are chickens. The satellite dish didn't make it in the move, and some time is spent playing board games rather than just watching TV. There isn't the money that there used to be, but there are not the same things to spend it on or the desire to spend it in the same way.

The everyday things go on, work is 9-5, but never at evenings or weekends. Dipping into community life offers rewards previously unrealised. Life is slower, there is more time to do the good things and although life may be quite hard at times the thought of accelerating back up to third or fourth gear is generally not even a consideration.

These people no longer valued what their previous life offered them, so the huge life swap was almost a release. They were not happy, their motivations had changed and so, they really were 'up for' trying something new. They love living a more simple life. They may miss the money from the old days, but they enjoy the compensations that their new life gives them.

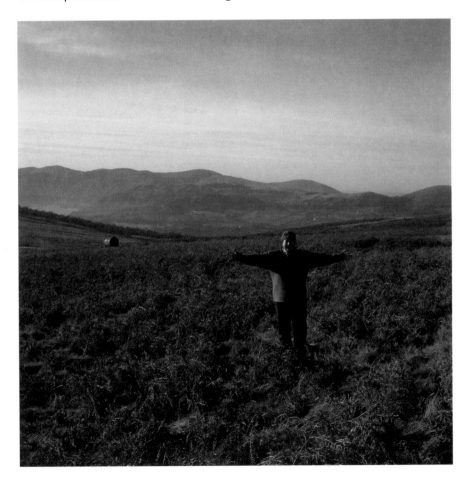

First gear

1 This is the big one! Here people have upped-sticks, left the job, sold the house, and moved to a completely new place . They have decided to go it alone. People who end up in this gear could be following their heart. They are impulsive.

They have grabbed life with two hands and are going to live it to the full. They want to fulfill their potential; achieve what they have always wanted to achieve; unleash their creativity; start all over again and go it alone.

They may start up a business, buy a business, work towards self-sufficiency, keep chickens, a goat and grow vegetables. The cupboards are full of home produce, the home-made wine is in the shed, the logs are collected, chopped and stacked by the back door and the brogues have been replaced by the wellies. This is a true life-swap. Ironically, people in this situation may work harder because the feeling of freedom and being in control of their own destiny really motivates them. They have definitely stepped off.

These people have little regard for security. However, the vast majority of people who downshift to this gear have money or savings behind them. They are risk takers, but they make sure that they calculate the risk. They know where the money is coming from. They may be good at planning and are confident in their own ability. A lot of people in this category end up cross-shifting where they swap their life, but end up working for themselves in a very successful business. They don't actually mind if things go wrong because they get a kick out of having tried, but they do work hard to succeed at the life swap.

Neutral

Lastly, there are those who simply get out of the car altogether. They leave life, as they have known it, behind. Sell up everything and move to live on a narrow boat or buy a camper van and drift around the world. They don't formally work and put all their money into buying and renovating a tumble down house. They just drop out completely and leave all they have known behind them.

If first gear people followed their heart then these people are the true romantics. They have scant regard for security or money. They will have understood what their needs will be in their new life and all they want is enough to live on. They may have money to finance the initial stages of the project, but no long term financial plans. They will confront the issue of having no money when the money runs out! They are confident that they can survive whatever life throws at them.

All six speeds have their own very unique appeal and there are pros and cons to living life in each of the different gears. It is about weighing up the good points and the bad points and working out for yourself which lifestyle suits you now and in the future.

Important Hint

Look at and talk to other people who have changed their lives to help you get some ideas about what gear and pace of life will suit you best.

Do you know what type of person you are?

The next step in planning your life swap is to try and analyse what sort of person you are. Some people make the mistake of leaping into a new life that they think will satisfy them only to find that they have completely the wrong sort of personality to be happy in that life.

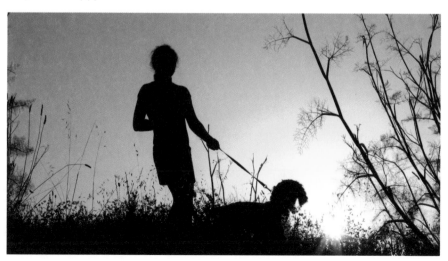

Personality types

The phrase 'personality type' is just another name for understanding what kind of person you are, what you thrive on and how you react in different situations.

'Some experts say that we develop our personality type throughout our early life.' It is in response to what happens in our lives, our environment and how things impact upon us. However, in later life, aspects of our personality once hidden can emerge. We start to question the things we have long felt comfortable with. Some of the less obvious aspects of our personality can become more dominant. Knowing who you are as a person is crucial to understanding what you want and need from your life in the future.

The leader: directs, delegates and inspires

Are you a natural manager who strives for efficiency? Do you enjoy thinking, planning and organising people to make improvements? Do you enjoy having the big ideas, but much prefer to leave the details to others?

If this is you, how will you find working for yourself? You are going to have the big ideas, but are you going to enjoy putting them into practice, especially when you have to design and complete the minute details of the project? Will you be happy being a leader without any followers?

The strategist: more theoretical than practical

Again, are you happier coming up with the ideas, but are likely to shy away from doing the accounts? Or will you become so wrapped up in future plans that you forget to pay the bills at all?

The nurturer: the people person

Are people more important to you than things? Would you be able to focus sufficiently on the task to succeed? Would you feel lonely and isolated if you started your own business as a one-person band? Are you in the sort of job now where you can nurture others and if not, is that contributing to why you want to swap?

The go-getter: creative, energetic and impulsive

Go-getters can sometimes put fun ahead of responsibilities, but they are flexible and have lots of energy. They enjoy learning new skills and could thrive working on their own project. However, they tend to have little regard for rules and can jump into situations without always thinking them through.

The idealist: committed to dreams, beliefs and aspirations

You live life on your own terms. Idealists don't always enjoy compromising, so if you are working for yourself then you will only have yourself to please. If you have been unhappy in your work because you felt you were always compromising your true values then swapping your life will be very liberating.

The resolver: the risk-taker

You enjoy taking a risk. You might find a life swap quite stimulating and enjoyable. However, you may not be the greatest decision-maker and may become cynical if you can't resolve situations quickly.

This is not the definitive list of personality types, but it gives some indications as to the different ways people behave and the differing ways people perceive opportunities or pitfalls.

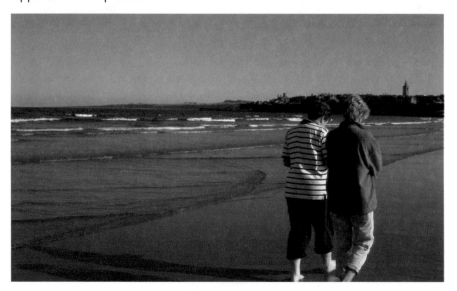

Stephanie

When Stephanie and her partner were considering downshifting, one of their options was to give up their jobs, sell up and go and live on a narrow boat. After some consideration, Stephanie thought that if she were going to give it all up she would rather go and live somewhere a bit warmer, but not too far away. She thought Spain would be good. It was warm, you could live quite cheaply and she decided that if they needed more money she could always go and stack shelves at the local supermarket. This idea was very attractive to them both, until one day when they were telling a friend about their plans, the friend laughed and said to Stephanie, "don't be ridiculous, you would hate it. Within three months you would be trying to manage the supermarket and in 12 months you would probably own it!"

This was a revelation for Stephanie. She had never really thought about what sort of person she was. She began to see that stepping off completely was not really an option for her. She is very driven. Stephanie is a leader and she would still need to to satisfy that part of her personality in her new life.

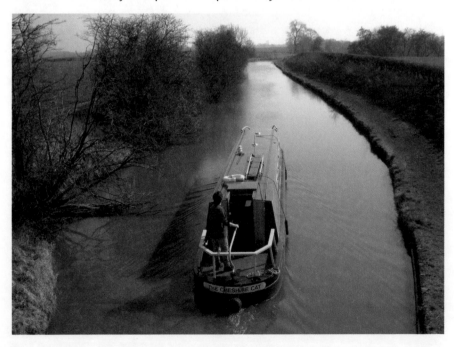

Step three: What kind of person are you?

This is a fun step. It will be useful to try and work out what makes you tick. What sort of things do you enjoy doing? Are you an extrovert? Are you a completer/finisher? Are you a perfectionist?

If you are contemplating a life swap, then you need to learn a little bit about yourself and your personality type. It is important to know what sort of life you will be happy living. You do not want to end up living a new life that drives you just as mad as the old one!

Activity

There are lots of books that have a personality test in them or you can find them on the Internet. Why not give one a go? This should not be an in-depth psychological analysis, just a thought-provoking exercise. Finding out what type of person you are, the attributes you have and what activities you enjoy doing, will help you to plan your future. Perhaps you will find that one of the reasons you are unhappy with your present life is because you are working in an environment that is at odds with your personality! Although it is really useful to be aware of your personality type, do not be restricted by the category and do not let it stop you doing something that you really want to do.

Important note: Not all psychologists agree on the different personality types or, in fact, that there are distinctive personality types.

Remember, there are lots of different ways in which you can satisfy your personality type. The leader, for example, may be very happy running their own business and working on their own without any staff to manage. They may satisfy the leadership part of their personality by doing some outside activity like being on the parish council or chairing the local amateur dramatics society.

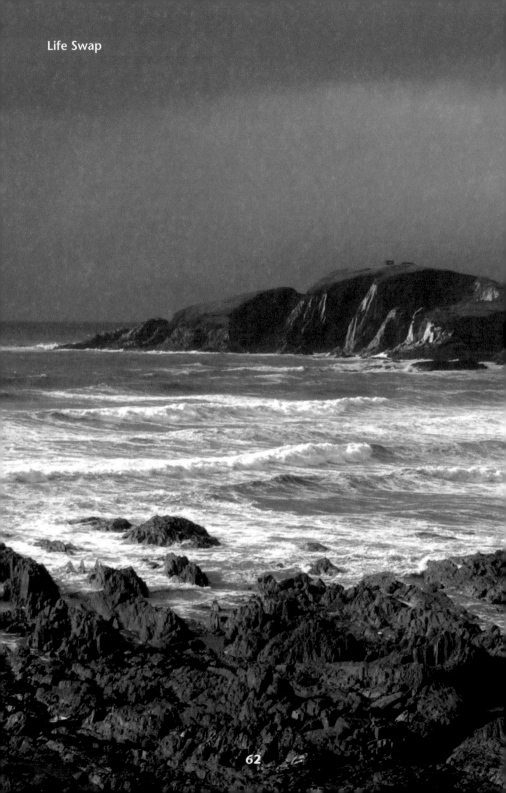

5

Discover what you want from your future

Perhaps the most important aspect of approaching a life change is to work out where you are going. It is not enough to know that you want to swap your life. You must work out what you want to swap it to.

There are endless stories of failed attempts at downshifting. Starting again is a HUGE step and it is vital to get it right. The cost of getting it wrong can be great, often leaving you in a worse situation than before. So the one thing that must be avoided, at all costs, is jumping out of the frying pan and into the fire.

" For every envy-inducing success story......there is a sorrier tale of downshifting moves that just don't work out" [10]

This is your opportunity to leave it all behind and start again. We have already looked at how you can analyse the bad bits, now you have to analyse what the good bits in your life are.

What do you want from your future?

Downshifting or planning a life swap is incredibly exciting. You have the opportunity to custom build your new life. There are no rights or wrongs when you are considering the life that you want to create for yourself, your partner and family. You need to identify all that is good in your present life.

Knowing what you don't want is only half the story. The other half is finding out what you do want. What do you want your new life to look like? What do you want to take with you from your present life and what do you want to leave behind?

(10) Red Magazine 2005

Step four:
The positives in your life

In this step, you are trying to identify the good things in your life that you want to take with you into your new life. Be honest here - this is about you and your future. It is about ensuring that you have a more satisfying and better quality of life. You don't want to throw the baby out with the bath water! Find the good things and make sure that you have them with you in your new life.

Activity

Take a good long look at the past 12 months.

• What was really good about it?

• What was it that made you happy?

• Make a list of all the good things in your life.

If you are fed up with not having enough time to enjoy your hobbies, then make sure you factor 'my time' into your new life. If you are fed up with commuting, try to make sure that you live near your work, or work from home. If never being around to see your children at the weekend frustrates you, then try to get a 9-5 job with weekends off and if you are fed up with your boss and always working towards someone else's goals, think about working for yourself.

In forcing yourself to analyse this, you will find out exactly what motivates you. In chapter three you identified the life-changing moments that ignited your dissatisfaction with life. Now we need to identify those moments in life that have made you feel really happy and in control.

Priorities and needs

When did you last think about what your priorities in life are? It isn't something that we normally spend a lot of time thinking about. However as we seize this fantastic opportunity to build a new life, we should make sure that the foundation is based upon our real priorities and needs.

Working out what your priorities in life are is not easy. It is very difficult to have any perspective on our own lives. We are often pulled from one direction to another and we are constantly trying to meet all of our obligations and responsibilities. It is no wonder that many of us rarely think about what is really important to us; what our real priorities in life are.

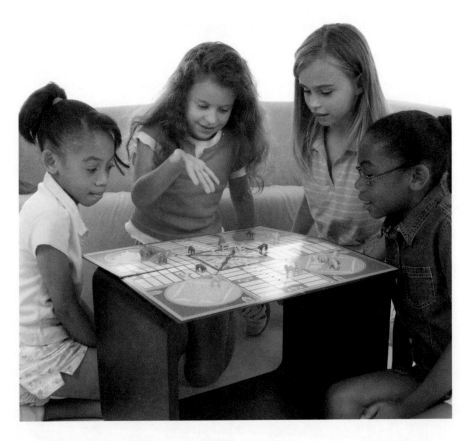

Step five: What is important to you?

Step five is probably the most important step. You need to make sure that your new life is built around the things that are really important to you – your life's priorities.

Activity

Take time to empty your mind for a few minutes and focus on your life and the activities and values that are important to you. Below is a suggested list but you may have other or more headings to add to it.

• Job	• Partner	• Career
• Children	• Money	• Hobbies
• Time for me	• Status	• Family
• House	• Leisure	• Friends
• Holidays	• Recognition	

1. Write down your own list of priorities.

2. Number them in priority order with 1 being the most important.

3. Take ten minutes to work out the approximate proportion of your life you spend on each priority. Write the percentage against each word.

4. Now compare the two.

Many people find that they spend most of their time on things at the middle to lower end of the list and least time on those priorities at the top of the list. This exercise will help you see what direction you want to take in your life. Some would say that family is their main priority, but when they really think about it they realise that they always miss their kid's football match and are never there to put them to bed.

Are you missing out on life?

Are you swept along by your life at such a pace that you don't have time to think about who you are, where you are, where you are going, and why?

Are there so many different facets to your life that you find yourself constantly being pulled in different directions and do not always know which are the really important ones? Are you constantly pressurised by the media, advertising, technology and science into a materialistic whirl that prevents you from stopping and looking at what is happening to your life?

Perhaps it is only on those rare occasions, when we stand still and assess our lifestyle that we question how we are living and why. Think back to your last two week holiday when your perspective slowly started to change. This was because you had the space to think. Your brain was not being assaulted for 10 hours a day about what you had to do.

> *"What is this life if, full of care,*
> *We have no time to stand and stare?"*
> *– Leisure, by W.H. Davies*

Tom

When Tom started thinking about his life and what his priorities were, he made an interesting discovery. He had listed his partner and children as his real priorities, but when he looked at his life he realised that he had been living as though his job and career were his main priority.

Tom also looked at what his needs were – what motivated him. He had a successful career and was a senior officer in the Police Service. He had moved his family around the country for promotion and was destined for the top of his profession.

To help him decide what his priorities were, Tom looked back to what motivated him to join the police initially and what he enjoyed about his work as a police constable. He enjoyed working independently as well as working as part of a close team, liked being outside and not in an office, interacting with people and not just doing paper work. He also enjoyed helping people and providing a good service. Although Tom now enjoys his job as a manager, it is a far cry from his life as a PC.

So now, twenty years on, although very successful he has begun to realise that the most obvious aspects of his current job - money, status and power/authority do NOT motivate him. And yet, here he is earning a lot of money. He is a leading member of his community and he is in charge of policing a large area of the county. But not one of these things fundamentally motivates him.

Tom was leading a busy life that appeared to be driven more by career and materialism than by personal and emotional fulfillment.

Are you caught in a trap?

How many of us are caught in the trap of living a life that we think we want? Or living a life we have drifted into rather than one we have consciously directed?

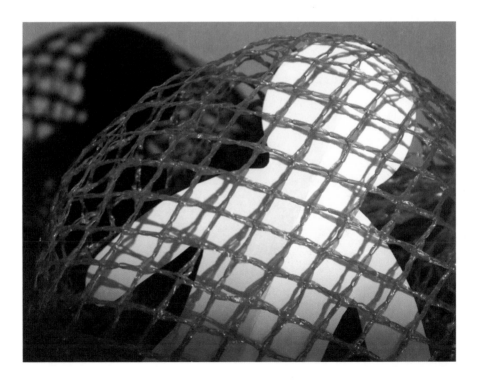

The five – question test

1. Is your life complicated and rushed?

2. Are you surrounded by possessions?

3. Do you hanker after a new car/camera/ television/outfit?

4. Do you have possessions/clothes/gifts that you have not looked at since you bought them?

5. Is your life everything you want it to be?

Look back to last Christmas or your last birthday. First of all, can you remember all the presents you received? How many of them did you want? More importantly, how many of them did you need? How many of them do you use/wear? Are any of them still in their packaging?

If you are contemplating changing your life or downshifting then one of the biggest steps you should consider taking before you make any decisions, is to work out what your life's 'needs' are as opposed to your life's 'wants'.

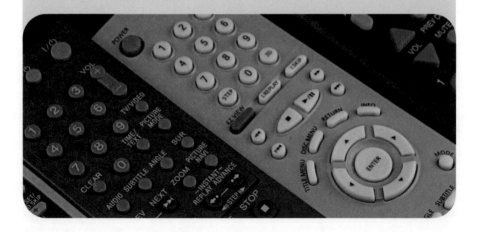

Step Six: Needs versus wants

In this step, you are trying to decide what are the essential things and what are the non-essential things in your life. Could you de-clutter? Could you throw out and live without all those possessions? How important are they to you? Could you live on much less money and still be happy?

Activity

Think about how you spend your money and what your spending patterns are. Do you spend for the sake of it? Do you surround yourself with material possessions? Could you do without them?

Make a list of your needs versus your wants. Write them down in two columns. Is a new car an essential or a non-essential in your new life? What about travel, new clothes, entertaining? Try and separate out what are the essentials you will need to live on.

It is OK for money and possessions to be important in your life. What is vital is that you work out what sort of lifestyle you will want to have because only then will you be able to calculate how much income you will need to sustain that lifestyle.

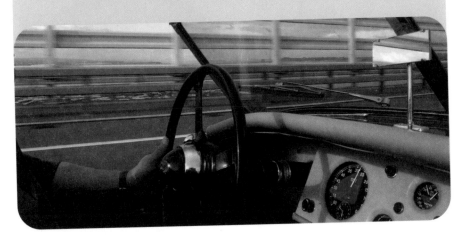

Mind swap

Downshifting is not just about moving house to a new location, or leaving your job and setting up on your own. There has to be some mental adjustment as well. If you just move your body and possessions to a new location without making some adjustment about the way you live and how you see your life, you could become just another unhappy statistic. Downshifting is the opportunity to make a fundamental change in your lifestyle. It is about much more than how you make a living or where you live. It is about HOW you live, about changing yourself to fit in with your philosophy of life and about getting back to basics. Living the life that is important to you, the life that YOU want to live, and not one you have drifted into. Who knows, you could achieve it without physically moving at all!

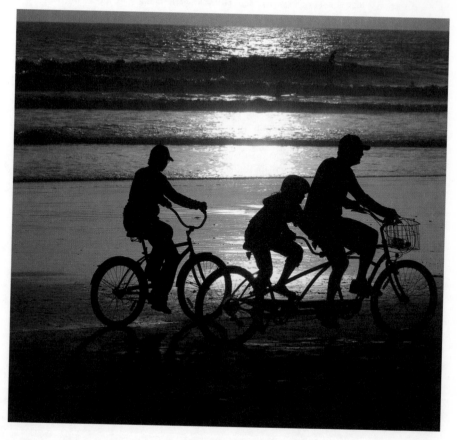

Ruth

Ruth used to live in the Southeast of England. Her husband was very successful; they lived in a large house and had a good standard of living. Ruth had a dream of moving to the country and leading a slightly different life. They decided to go into business together and so, she and her husband gave up their life in the Southeast and moved north to start again. They rented a large house in a village and started their new life. They both found working for themselves hard and four years later, they were still really missing the financial security of their past life.

"How I long for those glory days of 2000 when we had money"
– a comment from Ruth

Ruth is unhappy. One of the main reasons for this is that she has not made any fundamental mental adjustment to her new life. She has moved location and is doing different things, but in her mind she still wants to live the way she lived before.

Ruth is motivated by the trappings of success. She likes status. With hindsight, she now thinks that although she was happy being a medium-sized fish in a medium-sized pond, one of her reasons for moving was to achieve an even greater status in a smaller community. If you refer back to the activity of listing your priorities on page 67 you can see how this could have helped Ruth.

There are no rights or wrongs to downshifting, it doesn't matter whether you enjoy status or money as long as you recognise that you do and make sure that you are able to satisfy and sustain these wants in your new life.

Ruth's unhappiness could have been avoided had she spent enough time thinking through what type of person she is; what her priorities and needs are; where she was in her life, where she wanted to be and why, before she made the leap.

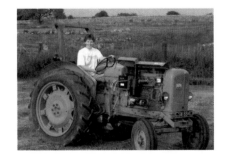

Phil

Phil is a great example of someone who made the necessary mental adjustments before downshifting. He made sure that he knew the sort of life he wanted to lead, how much money he would need and how he was going to make that money.

Phil used to have a highly-paid job. For many years, he worked and lived in fifth gear; buying a new car every two years. He loved cars and having the latest fast car was a reflection of his status and successes in life. But eventually, his pace of life became too much and he needed to make a change. Deep down, he had always dreamt of living the good life.

It was very clear to Phil that he had to change his views about his fast, hectic and materialistic lifestyle.

Four years ago, Phil downshifted with his family to a rural area. He now leads a completely different life to the one he used to lead. Does he miss his cars? "Yes" he said "sometimes, but I now have an old Land Rover and I love it, even when it lets me down! The best bit about it is that it cannot be mended by plugging it into a computer to diagnose the problem; you have to get inside the thing to find out what is wrong. This is how I used to maintain my cars when I was young."

When asked if he was happy Phil said " Yes, very. I don't really want for anything these days" he added, "but I do know that I have changed my 'wants'".

Phil has completely changed his outlook. He has adjusted his mind-set about what he wants out of life. He no longer craves the trappings of material success and he now gets pleasure out of very different things. Maintaining his own vehicle is immensely satisfying and more fun then booking it into a garage and being charged a fortune to have something done that he enjoys doing himself.

So how do you make sure that you are successful in your life swap like Phil and do not make the same mistakes as Ruth? It is about being brutally honest with yourself, your partner and your family about what you want from your new life and why.

Let's go back and check all the steps so far

Have you:

1. Pinpointed the areas in your life that are causing you unhappiness?

2. Analysed your life-changing moments and identified what you don't like about your life?

3. Thought about what personality type you might be and what future life will suit you best?

4. Identified what is good in your life now that you want to keep with you in the future?

5. Thought about what is really important in your life and what your priorities and values are?

6. Worked out your wants versus your needs and listed what is essential and non-essential in your life?

Once you have done all of this then you will be in a really good position to make some sound decisions about your new life – remembering all the time that downshifting is a life change and that the change has to take place in the mind as well as in the body.

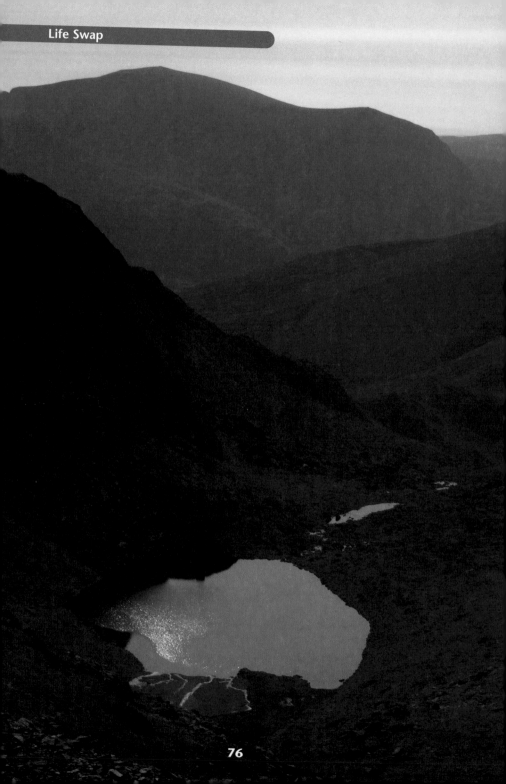

6

Reality check – the downside of downshifting

It is wonderful to have a dream and the dream of stepping off the treadmill and opting for a simpler life is one that thousands of people share. Not everyone will do something about trying to realise their dream and even those that do will often find that the reality is somewhat different from the dream.

Downshifting is a huge move and can be a risky business, but there are a number of things that can be done to minimise the risks. The most important of which is to identify some of the things that can go wrong and either work to avoid them or prepare for them.

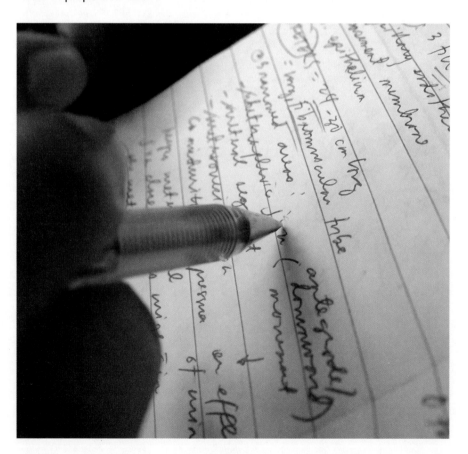

Step Seven: Your approach to a life swap

This step is a very useful way of identifying how you might approach your life swap. Again, it is a way of minimising the stress and trauma of living through a major change.

Activity

Spend a little time looking back to a time when you lived through a change – it can be anything – from changing job to moving house, or leaving school or college.

Then think about these questions:

1. How did you cope with it?

2. What aspect of it was most challenging?

3. How did you behave towards your friends/colleagues/partner/family during the change?

4. How did they behave towards you?

5. What could you have done differently to reduce the stress of the change?

Write down your answers.

Very few big changes in life are simple or easy and it is useful to think about how you cope generally with 'change' in your life. Understanding and anticipating some of the issues that have affected you in the past may help you to minimise the impact they have on you in the future.

Beware of doubts

The impact of leaving your comfort zone can be difficult to deal with, not just physically, but emotionally as well.

Often, when people are thinking about moving out of their comfort zone – i.e. when they are thinking about a life swap or change – something quite interesting happens. Subconsciously, they sabotage their own ability to embark on that change. They skillfully manage to talk themselves out of doing it, and come up with every reason why they shouldn't make the change.

This process can happen both internally and externally. Firstly, they begin to have doubts about making the change. Nagging doubts surface about why the move will not work and why the risk is too great. They begin to lose confidence and doubt their own ability to succeed. Instead of being excited, they become more and more anxious about taking the risk.

Doubts like -

"What happens if I fail?"

"I don't have the skills to start my own business!"

"Who would want to buy my paintings anyway?"

"I don't know how to keep chickens"

"The job I have now is safe"

"I need my savings for a rainy day"

"I will miss the city"

"What about my pension?"

...etc

All of these are obvious doubts when approaching a life change but some are more relevant or sensible than others. Many people, instead of working through all these doubts and putting them into some sense of proportion, actually let them take over. They hide behind these fears and let them sabotage their confidence, destroy their enthusiasm and stop them moving towards a better life.

The external process can be even more debilitating. It happens when those people around you start giving you advice as to why you should not change your life. Often, this is for their own reasons. It could be because they are jealous of what you are trying to achieve or perhaps they don't have the courage to do it themselves. They may have an inner need to maintain the status quo and are frightened of change. Maybe what you are contemplating is beyond their comprehension or perhaps they just don't want you to move away. If you ever smoked, do you remember giving 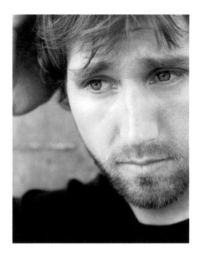 up? Smokers will always try and get you back in their club. You giving up calls into question their own lives. Conformity is the whole premise upon which society rests.

When things change around you it can be unsettling, almost frightening; your safe little world can seem threatened. There is enormous pressure put on us to conform and not rock the boat. People feel safe and secure in familiar surroundings. They, often, don't want to venture into places that are new and they certainly don't want you to go there.

You will hear comments like –

"Are you mad – look at what you will be losing"

"You can't do that"

"What do you know about running your own business?"

"Do you know how hard it is to work for yourself?"

"You will never be happy in the country"

"Your home is here – with us"

"You'll never do it"

...etc

Step eight: Doubts, panics & problems

If you don't identify what it is that has been stopping you from swapping your life, you will never be able to get past it and therefore, will never be able to change. So this one is important. You need to recognise that you are having these doubts and that they are coming from inside you. Once you know what they are, you can begin to deal with them and get on with planning your new life. You also need to identify those people around you who are sapping your strength and confidence.

Activity

Every time a doubt comes into your mind, a panic, a problem, or a voice that says you cannot make this move, write it down. Think about it rationally. Is it a sensible and practical problem? If it is, think about how you will solve it. If it is irrational then put it out of your mind.

Now write down a list of the people who are against your change and who are trying to talk you out of it. Try and distance yourself from these people. It will be hard enough coping with your own doubts without having them reinforced by those around you.

Surround yourself with people who are 'in your corner', those who are encouraging in their comments, who admire your courage, who are as excited as you are by the opportunity you are creating for yourself, and who give you confidence; not the jealous people who want you to fail.

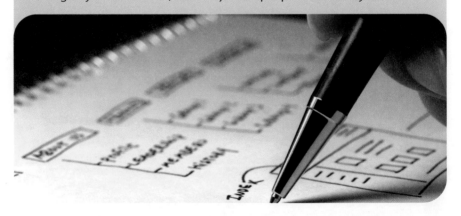

Money

Money is inevitably one of the biggest issues in downshifting particularly when we look at the pressure on all of us to ensure our own financial security.

Downshifting by definition means living a simpler life. Generally, you do not need as much money to live a simpler life and more often than not, people find themselves living on greatly reduced incomes once they have downshifted – at least initially.

Whist this is a rather obvious point, the loss of security and the absence of the pay cheque every month can be hard to come to terms with.

A recent look at downshifting shows that while 34% of people are happy with downshifting and don't miss their previous income, 38% are happy with downshifting but do miss their previous income, and 16% although still happy, found the drop in income very hard. [11]

Mourning the loss of income and lifestyle can completely destroy all the benefits of downshifting and cause people to be unhappier in their new life than they were in their old life. This is the reason why there needs to be a mental adjustment to how you live in your new life, as well as a physical one. If you are going to downshift, it is important to plan your finances very carefully. Try and get some financial advice, but be aware that many financial advisors will try and stop you downshifting. They want to advise you to earn more, save more, build your pension, buy bonds, buy unit trusts, invest etc. The last thing they want you to do is lower your income. It is important to have some money behind you or some earning capacity early on in your new life. Changing your life will initially cost you money and these costs can be considerable.

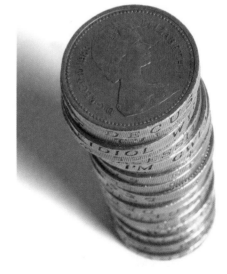

(11) Downshifters Retrospective Reflections
   – Australia Institute

Look at the cost of moving house:

- Solicitor's fees
- Surveyor's fees
- Storage costs
- Estate agent fees
- Removal costs
- Stamp duty if you are buying another house

And that is before you move in!

Some people minimise the risk of downshifting by keeping their house and renting it out, whilst at the same time renting a smaller house in the new location. This means that if it all goes wrong you have something to move back to, but it also generates income that may cover your new rent and give you a small amount left over every month.

Once you have moved in, there may be the cost of some new furniture, white goods or decorating to be done. Work to be done on the garden can be expensive. If you are going to be growing vegetables and fruit there is the start-up costs of plants, seeds and trees – all of which will take several months or years to become established enough for you to start reaping the benefits. Then there are the new school uniforms for the children and new clothes more suitable for outdoor living. And you may want to factor in some money to enable you to take a holiday in the first 12 months – because you will need it!

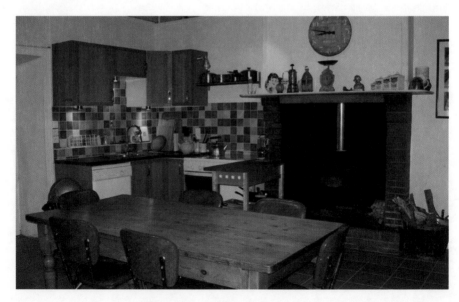

Step nine: Budgeting

In step six you will have identified what your wants are as opposed to your needs. In this step you need to look at your list of needs and try and calculate an approximate amount of money you will need for each one. Then you can start to fill out a cash flow forecast for the first 12 months of your new life.

Activity

Spend some time looking at your spending patterns. Try to plan how much money you need to live on, taking into consideration how much it costs you to live and work where you are now. Remember it costs money to go to work – travel, work clothes, bought lunches, equipment etc. – expenses that may now have gone or have been greatly reduced.

Once you know how much you will need to live on, you can work out how long you could survive without a full-time income and how long you could survive on a part-time income or savings.

A simple cash flow forecast might help you with your budgeting.

Tim and Susan

Have a look at the chart on the next page. This is a simple process that Tim and Susan went through to see how much they would need to live on in their new life.

They decided that they would rent their old house out for the first 12 months of their life swap. Their dream was that both Tim and Susan would become self-employed, working in their areas of expertise. Tim wanted to give up his office job and start a web design business. Susan wanted to give up her teaching career and concentrate on privately teaching music.

They had £15,000 of savings and they were going to use that to live off until they built up their businesses.

Income	Oct	Nov	Dec	Jan	Feb	March	April	May	June	July	Aug	Sep	TOTAL
Savings	1,200	1,200	1,200	1,200	1,200	1,200	1,200	1,200	1,200	1,200	1,200	1,200	14,400
Rent	200	200	200	200	200	200	200	200	200	200	200	200	£2,400
P.O.			£1,000	£1,500									£2,500
M income				£500	£500	£500	£250	£500	£500	£500		£500	£3,750
C income				£250	£300	£500	£500	£500	£500	£500	£250	£750	£4,050
Total income	£1,400	£2,400	£2,900	£2,150	£2,200	£2,400	£2,150	£2,400	2,400	£2,400	£1,650	£2,850	£27,100
Expenditure													
Rent	£500	£500	£500	£500	£500	£500	£500	£500	£500	£500	£500	£500	£6,000
Food	£200	£400	£400	£400	£400	£400	£400	£400	£400	£400	£400	£400	£4,600
Petrol	£100	£100	£100	£100	£100	£100	£100	£50	£100	£100	£200	£100	£1,250
Insurance	£450												£450
Insurance	£35	£35	£35	£35	£35	£35	£35	£35	£35	£35	£35	£35	£420
Car		£160						£280					£440
Holiday								£500			£500		£1,000
Utilities	£120	£120	£120	£120	£120	£120	£120	£120	£120	£120	£120	£120	£1,440
C Tax	£70	£70	£70			£70	£70	£70	£70	£70	£70	£70	£700
Uniform	£150											£150	£300
Plants	£200				£50			£50					£300
Incidentals	£200	£200	£200	£200	£200	£200	£200	£200	£200	£200	£200	£200	£2,400
Total	£2,025	£1,425	£1,585	£1,355	£1,355	£1,475	£1,705	£1,925	£1,425	£1,425	£2,025	£1,575	£19,300.00
Total	-£625	£975	£1,315	£795	£845	£925	£445	£475	£975	£975	-£375	£1,075	£7,800
C'rrd f'wrd	-£625	£350	£1,665	£2,460	£3,305	£4,230	£4,675	£5,150	£6,125	£7,100	£6,725	£7,800	
Savings left													£7,800

They had been going to give themselves four months to settle in and get used to their new surroundings, but Tim managed to get a temporary job with the Post Office over the Christmas period and that really helped them.

In budgeting, they pulled right back and decided to live a very economical life until they knew how much they would be earning. They looked at the essential expenditure for the year and added a small amount for extras which would include the occasional visit to the cinema, a meal out or extra on food.

Pulling right back on expenditure was quite a shock for them, but it really helped them to sort out their wants from their needs and also ensured that when the income started coming in, they began to enjoy a few treats. This also allowed them to be confident about the minimum amount they needed to live on, in case one of their businesses did not provide the anticipated income.

They factored in some money to have a break away after a few months and then another week camping with the children in the summer holiday. Susan only taught in the school term time and Tim worked from home helping other small businesses with their web sites. As their income increased, they relied less and less on their savings, enabling them to put some money back to help with the eventual house sale/purchase or for an emergency like major car expenditure.

This is a very simple example, but it shows how very careful planning and budgeting is essential to helping you to succeed.

Relationships

Personal relationships can suffer when you live in the fast lane. There never seems to be enough time to spend with the people that matter. You hardly see your partner and are more like ships passing in the night!

However, living through a life change can also put a huge strain on relationships. Especially when partners have rubbed along very well, busy in their own separate work-filled lives. Even though partners go through a life change together, they may react very differently to it. It can be hard to offer support to your partner when you are having difficulty adjusting yourself. They may want different things.

> *"Make sure your relationship is strong enough to cope with the changes, stresses and strains"*
> – advice from Helen at La Maison Rose (see case study on pg. 126).

The stress levels may be high, particularly in the early days and working to support and reassure each other is important.

Relationships with family and friends may suffer as well. You may lose some of those friends who were negative about your move just because you distanced yourself from them and their negative attitudes.

Richard

Richard said that one of the reasons he downshifted was because he no longer had time for family and friends. Now he has much more time to see them.

The bit he hadn't factored in was that they haven't downshifted, are still living in the fast lane, and do not have time to see him.

It may be hard when you are learning to live on your now small income, to hear about past friends and colleagues getting promotions, moving to bigger houses or retiring on large pensions. It is important, at this point, to remind yourself of why you downshifted and look at the benefits. One tip is to imagine being asked to return to your old job. Would you do it? I suspect not! Having decided that, it is easier to look at how good your life is now and not think about others.

Children

Do not expect all children to be as thrilled and excited at the prospect of a life swap as you are! Not all of them will view it as a positive thing. Teenagers, in particular, may find a move very disrupting, especially if they get moved to a rural location just as they are beginning to enjoy the social aspect and amenities of urban living.

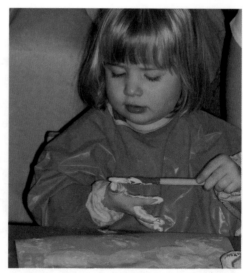

It can also be disruptive if they have to move school and make new friends. Some will find this easier than others; some will hate it and rebel and not be at all receptive to, or appreciative of, the benefits of their new existence. For these reasons, the decisions being taken about a life swap have to be made after full discussions with all family members. All thought processes should be shared with the children. Lets look at it from their perspective.

To them it may mean:

- Leaving their home
- Fewer friends
- Losing their old friends
- Moving to a new school
- Less family money
- Less excitement
- Less to do
- Less activities close by

- Being more dependant on parents for transport

- More supervision and involvement from parents who will be around more now.

Selling the benefits of a family life swap to the younger members of the family may be one of the hardest parts of downshifting.

Working for yourself

Think about whether you are the right sort of person to work for yourself. This life does not suit everyone. Go back to step three on page 61 and check out what personality type you are. How will working for yourself fit in with who you are as a person?

Some people will feel very isolated and vulnerable working for themselves, especially if you are used to working in a big organisation. Those people who are sociable and enjoy working in a team or with others may find working on their own very lonely and will crave outside stimulation.

It is much easier to work for someone else. You don't have the responsibility and if you don't like what is happening at work you can blame the 'management'. When you work on your own, there is no one else to blame. When you want support and reassurance that you are doing the right thing, there is no one to give it. And some people just do not like the pressure of running their own business.

Important note

If you are the sort of person who suffers from bouts of ill health or you take a number of days off sick from work every year, then think very carefully before you start to work for yourself. Being ill, when you are self-employed, is simply not an option! As a retailer, when you have orders to get out and customers to satisfy and there is just you, or you and your partner to do it, being sick is very inconvenient and can cause lots of problems for the business. Of course, you can't help it when ill health strikes, but being physically and mentally strong and looking after yourself is vital.

Do not be under any illusions; you will work harder when you work for yourself than you have ever worked for anyone else.

Working for yourself has great benefits, but it is not always easy. The buck stops with you, you have total responsibility for the success of the business and if it goes wrong there is no one else to blame. You may be your own boss, but you have to make all the decisions. Of course, the reverse is also true, each and every success is yours!

Working together

Do not be lulled into the belief that working with your partner will be a romantic experience – it probably won't! The fantasy that many have of sitting on the bench outside their gallery and tea room watching the sun go down at the end of another enjoyable profitable day sipping wine is exactly that – a fantasy! The reality is much more likely to be that you haven't spoken for two days, you have been working for 14 hours, your partner is doing the bookkeeping and you have at least two more hours work to do before you can think about stopping.

Marie and Gwynn

Marie and Gwynn had given up their jobs in the Midlands and moved up North to start their own business. They were very excited about their new life. They sold their house, bought a smallholding and embarked upon starting their own business and building their dream. Their two children were equally as excited with their move to the country.

The first 6 months went very well, but by the time they had been there a year Marie and Gwynn were in separate bedrooms. They were working together and living together. They were trying to learn new skills, did not have a lot of money and they argued about the business. Gwynn was used to making decisions at work, but Marie challenged his decisions because she felt that she had an equal right in the decision-making process – after all it was her business too. They rowed, cried and screamed. They didn't speak to each other for days at a time and they were both really regretting the move.

The children were unhappy because they were living in an atmosphere of continual friction and arguments and Marie felt that her world was coming to an end.

There are a number of things that you can do to prevent this from happening or to help you cope with it when it does happen.

First of all, think about your days off. When things were going badly for Marie and Gwynn, they thought that they needed some quality time together, so they would go out on their day off together and argue! Actually, what they really needed was time away from each other. Eventually, they used to take days off separately and go and do their own thing. It is almost impossible to live and

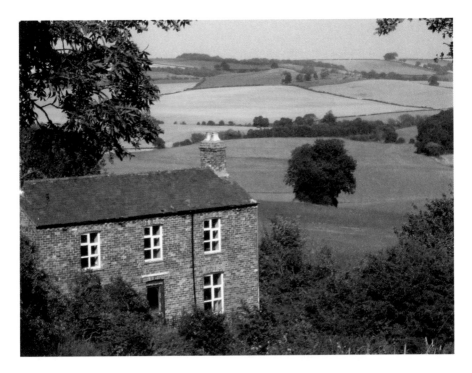

work with the same person all day, every day and still expect to get on well. You need a break from each other.

Secondly, they divided the workload to play to each others skills and strengths. Even though both partners ran the business, they tried to divide the areas of work. Gwynn looked after the purchasing and production and Marie looked after the sales and marketing. They still had a say in each other's area, but they no longer felt they both needed to control the whole of the business. They split the responsibility, lessened their workload and lowered their stress. They started getting on better.

Two years on, they are much happier as a family and the business is going well. Their story is by no means the exception. Many couples go through a similar experience as they adjust to their new life together.

The secret is to know that this may happen and not to despair when it does. If it gets bad, talk to others who have been through the experience and see how they coped.

Skills base

One of the reasons that a number of small businesses fold in the first three years of trading (between 30 – 40% according to many sources) is because the people running them do not have the right skills.

'Downshifters' are sometimes guilty of this. One of the reasons for this is that as part of the move to start again, they leap into the unknown and opt to do something completely different with their lives. Often, they turn to a hobby or a lifelong ambition on which to base their new venture.

In making this transition, they run the risk of turning their back on many of the skills that they have amassed throughout their working life.

Be careful if you decide to go it alone – if you have been used to working in a team you might find it isolated and lonely. And, if you are in a very social working environment where you are constantly dealing with people, you might hate working from home.

If you have always worked in a service industry and have not been used to business management or accounting you might find book-keeping, tax, VAT and budgeting for your business very stressful.

If you have been used to an office job and you move to fulfill your creativity by becoming a crafts person, you may be very good at your craft, but not so good at selling or marketing.

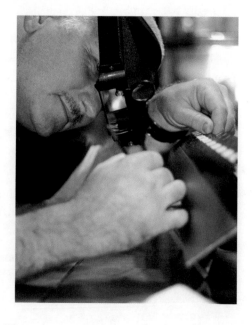

Likewise, if you are used to working on your own much of the time you may find it difficult to go into a retail business where you have to deal with staff, complaints and customer service all day! And if you have worked as part of a team, you may find employing and managing staff difficult.

Alan

Alan had worked in social services for over twenty years. He decided that the job he had signed up for had changed dramatically. He was now spending his time doing paperwork, complying with increased rafts of legislation and trying to hit performance targets. He decided to give it all up and start again. He had quite a lot of money saved and he thought that he would buy a small rural business.

He came across a small fish farm that was for sale in Scotland. Alan had always enjoyed fishing and he thought that this was right up his street. Within 12 months the business was failing. Alan may have enjoyed fishing, but he knew very little about running a business and even less about hatching and keeping fish.

Alan's real skills were with people. He had great communication skills, great interpersonal skills and an aptitude for working with and helping others. The dream of the fish farm was very different to the reality. He found that he was lonely working on his own and he didn't like all the paperwork and book-keeping. Working with the environmental health officers and Defra was as much of a nightmare for him as his social work job had been before.

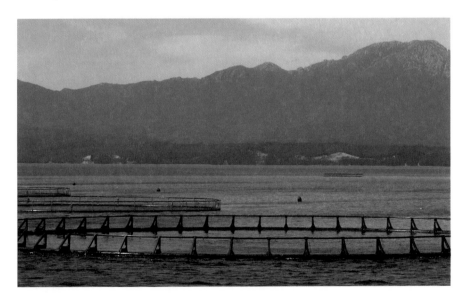

Rae

Rae was worried that she would never be able to get a job when her children left home. She said she hadn't really got any skills because she hadn't ever had a proper job. The only thing she had been was a part-time Tupperware lady.

When asked what that had entailed, she said that she had to cook meals that Tupperware products could be used for. Then she had to go out and find people who would host a party. At the party she gave a presentation about the products showing, through her recipes and food, how she had used them. After that she took orders for the items. At home she ordered the items, sent the invoices, arranged the deliveries and collected the money.

No skills! We just laughed. Rae was immensely skilled. Quite apart from the huge amount of skill she had to have to run a home and family, just look at all the other skills she had to have to perform the Tupperware job:

- Influencing skills
- Interpersonal skills
- Communication skills
- Research skills for suitable recipes
- Cooking skills
- Marketing skills
- Selling
- Public speaking
- Presentation skills
- Administration skills
- Logistics
- Finance skills
- Customer service

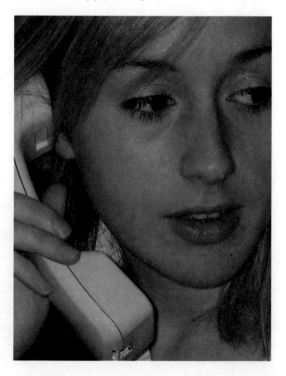

Step ten: Skills assessment

In this step we ask you to look at your skills base. It is useful here to think about basic skills that you have – the ones that you don't really think about or that you take for granted like communication skills.

Activity

• Make a list of all the jobs you have had since you left school.

• Write down against each job, the skills you think you needed to do it and the skills you learnt by doing it.

• If you haven't been employed, but have spent time running a family or household, write down the skills you feel you have used whilst doing this.

• Look at the list. Many of those skills will be transferable and will be very useful in any other work that you have in the future. This list will help you to plan any future employment or business. Look at the competencies you will need or that the employers are asking for and then look at your list. You might be surprised!

Cross-shifting

The other side of the coin are those people who downshift to start their own venture and within a few short years have built up a thriving business.

Many of these people haven't in fact downshifted, they have cross-shifted. This means that although they have undergone some changes in their lives, either they have re-located or started up on their own, they still find that they are working harder than they ever did before, with long hours, some stress and little leisure time. And they are making just as much money as they did before - if not more.

The one upside of this is that unlike their previous life, they are working to their own goals, they are in control of their lives and everything they do is for themselves. Workaholics – beware this trap! Make sure you know what you really want out of your future before you make the leap. If working less is one of your goals then keep a tight rein on the amount of work you take on and put more of your energy into your hobbies and leisure time.

Moving to the country

How many times have you been on holiday and ended up gazing into estate agents' windows dreaming of living there? This can be a big mistake because the stress free atmosphere of being on holiday may be far removed from the reality of living and working in that location.

The lure of the country idyll may be strong to those living in an urban area, but beware of being sucked into it. Country life can be hard. Nothing is around the corner like in the city. Public transport may be scarce, if it exists at all. If you are used to 24 hour shopping, a good public transport system, cultural venues, better public services, hospitals and schools nearby then you may be in for a shock. As we have said before, sometimes these differences are harder for children to come to terms with than their parents.

Do not expect to be welcomed with open arms. The people living in the country may not always appreciate the city dwellers coming in and buying up all the best properties. There may be a feeling that with all the 'incomers', the fabric of their community is being eroded, and fitting in may be difficult at first. Unlike the anonymity of city life, nothing much goes unnoticed in a village. You may not like the loss of anonymity or the feeling that you are living in a goldfish bowl.

Employment

If you are thinking of downshifting to a simpler life in a rural area and plan to find a job when you get there, it is worth doing a lot of research into what job opportunities there are before you make any significant decisions. Generally, there are not the same employment opportunities in rural areas as there are in towns or cities. In addition, the jobs that are available are unlikely to offer the same remuneration as you could expect to earn in the city.

In this chapter, we have looked at some of the pitfalls of downshifting.

It is important not to be put off by the things mentioned above. Think about them, prepare for them and embrace them as part of the challenge.

7

Dream on – the upside of downshifting

Regaining control

Living through a life swap gives you the opportunity to create time and regain control of your life. Think about having complete control over your day, making your own decisions and having time to do what you want to do.

Can you imagine a life where:

- You make all the decisions

- You have time to do what you want to do

- You answer to no one but yourself

- Your travelling is not controlled by rush hour traffic

- You can factor into your timetable one part of every week as 'your time'

- You decide what meetings you want or need to go to

- You work as hard or not as you want or are able to

- You can make a decision to take on a contract or not – depending on your money/leisure situation at that time

- You can work late some evenings and leave early the next

- You can plan to go out or entertain during the week

- If things are getting too hectic you can cut down on work

- You are in control

- You have enough time.

An overriding sense of freedom

Although some people who downshift may end up working harder than they did before, it is a different sort of work, with completely different pressures and stresses. And because it is you making the decisions, the impact of these stresses tends to be far less negative and can, frequently, be positive.

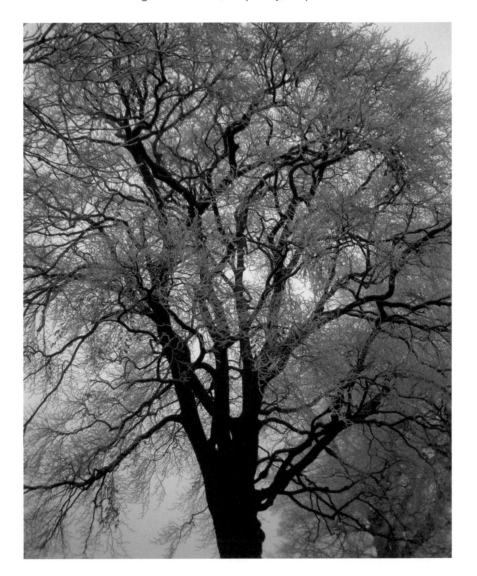

Joe and Rosemary

Having worked in an office for the previous 10 years, it was an amazing feeling for Joe and Rosemary to suddenly find themselves running their own business. The business premises they found were two large rooms that had been restored from an old stable block in a stately home. Joe and Rosemary said that one of the best things for them about working for themselves was being able to get into work early, make a good start and then at 10.30 every morning, make coffee and go and sit out on the grass. There were red squirrels and hares and they could hear woodpeckers and see buzzards flying overhead. Everyday, they thought how lucky they were. When Rosemary thought of their past friends and colleagues battling with city living she would laugh and say "If only they could see us now."

Joe and Rosemary worked in the tourist industry and still worked seven days a week for part of the year, but it was for themselves and they were in control of what they did and how they did it. There were busy times and less busy times. In the less busy times, they took half days and enjoyed leisure pursuits. Joe went fishing and Rosemary walked. When they were busy, they put all their efforts into the business and enjoyed it more because it was their decision to do so. It was up to them how they planned their work and leisure time.

They felt totally in control of their new life and they had control of their time. They still worked hard to get their business going, but they had created time and that time allowed them to play hard as well as work hard. They now had a much more fulfilling life.

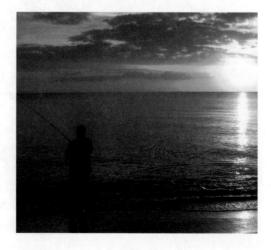

This sense of freedom often comes with an empowering sense of responsibility. You can do what you want, make the decisions and take responsibility for the consequences. This is liberating. This is your life. You are living life at your own pace.

Regain your social life

This sense of regaining control is not confined just to work. It applies to your social life as well. In your new life, you have managed to create more leisure time to do the things you enjoy, whether its going to the cinema, having friends around for supper or going for a long walk. For the first time in years, social occasions are not confined to weekends and you can socialise with true friends – not colleagues who you felt you should spend time with. You now control your working day and you have more flexibility to free up time when it suits you.

Job Satisfaction

Whether you start your own business, do voluntary work, buy a business or go to work for someone else, your new working environment should be very different from the old one.

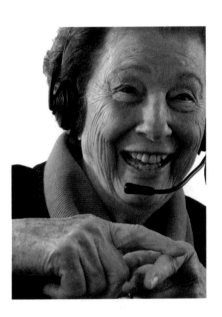

Swapping to a simpler life should give you the opportunity to work in an environment that suits you better. There should be less stress or only stress at a level that you can happily manage. You should be able to create more time for other pursuits and activities and you should be working on your own terms, not someone else's.

Voluntary Work

There are those who embark on a life swap who don't want to re-start their work or career. They may be looking for local part-time work or even unpaid activities. This can be an opportunity to do something stimulating and rewarding without the full responsibility of a paid job. Being able to put something back into the community can satisfy all sorts of 'service' needs in people. Often, as part of your new life or even following retirement, there is enjoyment to be had in taking on positions within the community. These can be really demanding and completely different from anything you have known before.

Working for yourself

If you work for yourself then the satisfaction levels should be great.

There are no more bosses, no more working to other people's goals or deadlines. Even though you may be on your own and having to make some hard decisions, you are the boss. You work in the knowledge that you will reap the benefit of all your labours. There is no more being let down by others lack of motivation.

Running your own business gives you freedom. It is a motivating experience that can be exciting, exhilarating and satisfying especially when you know that every achievement is yours to savour.

Just being able to think positively about your future is very powerful and motivating. How much better to be able to plan your own work and determine where you business will go over the next 12 months, rather than worrying about when you might get the next promotion, whether you have to apply for your own job after the re-structuring, or how you will manage to find the time to study for an exam or assessment.

There may of course be a level of stress that goes with this life choice. The responsibility of running your own business can be scary, but it is all part of the exhilaration. It is a different sort of stress and is easier to manage because everything else seems so new and exciting. Manageable stress is actually part of the excitement and a powerful motivator. "Enjoy the fear!"

"We can honestly say that moving from our jobs and lives in London was one of the best decisions we have ever made. That's not to say the decision - or our lives here - have been easy! The work has been hard, at times seemingly impossible. But every achievement has been so satisfying" – a comment from Simon at Augill Castle (see case study on pg. 121).

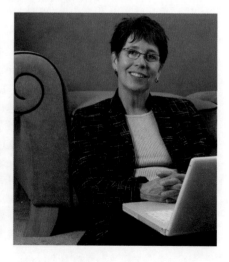

Health

Remember, there is little point in swapping your life unless you are changing to a better quality of life. Swapping to a simpler life really should go hand in hand with being able to lead a healthier life.

The world certainly does look a rosier place when you free yourself from the shackles of a life you were unhappy leading. This may in itself mean you are healthier. You should also feel happier, calmer and more content.

It is important to look after yourself and keep healthy if you are going to be self-employed. Being physically and mentally fit has great benefits and will help you, generally, have a better sense of well-being. Being in control, and having time for yourself helps you create a positive mental attitude towards your work and your life and this in turn is important to maintaining good health.

Those people who decide to downshift to a more rural area should also reap the benefits of cleaner and less polluted air.

Exercise

If you are managing to work fewer hours or are in control of the hours you work, you may be able to factor in a period of exercise on a regular basis. If you are working from home, it is especially important to find the time to get out of the working environment – your house – to have a break and take some exercise.

One of the challenges people face when working from home is finding the discipline to develop a work routine. This can be as much about shutting the office door at 5pm and not working through the evening as it is about having regular breaks and exercise. Most importantly, if you are working in a less stressful environment with more control over your time then hopefully, the hurried sandwich on the run or the chocolate bar as a meal substitute will disappear and be replaced with a proper break and more nourishing meals.

Working in a less built up area may allow the family to get out more. Children can play out with other children in the village more than they could in an urban area. Whilst you may not be near big sporting venues and other entertainment centres, there are still other activities for children and adults that can lead to more of a focus on participating in activities like walking, sailing, pony riding, choirs, orchestras, book clubs, local football leagues, village cricket teams etc.

Food

There is a great resurgence of good locally-produced food in most rural areas. There are not only farmers' markets which can be found all around the country, but also farm shops, local shops and producers selling their own goods, or organic produce sold at the farm gate. Interest in 'food miles', organic and non-GM produced foods is very much part of current debate and there is a growing trend for 'traceability' in food products, particularly in rural areas.

This new simple life should give you more time. If you are no longer dependent on supermarkets, convenience foods and services then you will have time to cook home-prepared food. Gone are the days of getting ready-made meals from the freezer or calling for a take-away. If you do get something out of the freezer, it is more likely to be the fresh vegetables or fruit from the garden that you froze last summer.

Healthcare

The term 'lottery' has been much used recently when referring to the level of healthcare provided in the UK. Whilst there may be endless reports on the availability of healthcare in different areas, it is generally assumed that access to a doctor at a smaller rural medical practice is easier than at a large urban medical practice, although medical facilities and specialist services may be further away and harder to reach.

Obviously, leading a simpler quieter way of life has general health benefits. If the quality of life improves, and people are happier, more positive and more content, it would not be unreasonable to hope that general health will improve and that they will rely less on healthcare services anyway.

Personal relationships

Personal relationships with family and friends may suffer in the fast lane. As we identified with Richard's case study in the last chapter, one of his reasons for downshifting was that he didn't feel as though he had free time to spend with his family and friends.

Time is the one investment that is needed to build and sustain personal relationships. As you lead this simpler life, you should have more time and more control over your time. Having time to build and sustain relationships must surely be one of the great benefits of swapping your life.

We have identified that relationships may not always be easy in the early days of a life swap, but even just being at home more allows you more time to spend with your partner and family. Even if relationships are not perfect, at least in your new life you will have some time to spend on improving them, rather than either being too busy or walking away from the relationship because it is too hard.

Friends

You will have the opportunity to improve your social life. There will be new friends to make and new relationships to build as you create a social circle. If you are a social person, put some effort into this aspect of your new life and really enjoy finding and cultivating new and stimulating friends.

Rural living can be very different from urban living. You may not have the same level of anonymity in a rural area and the sense of 'community' is often very different. For a lot of people, there is great satisfaction to be gained in participating actively in community life.

Children

Children are just as badly affected by life in the fast lane as adults. They sense the stress, tension and unhappiness. They want to see more of their parents and will resent the fact that their mother and father are always at work, or working in the evenings or at the weekends. It is important for all small children to feel that they are at the centre of their parents immediate world and often, in the long hours culture, this may not be the case.

A BBC Panorama programme in early 2006 asked children what they thought about their parents working such long hours. The general consensus of opinion was that "they (their parents) should get a life"! – 'Out of the mouths of babes....!'

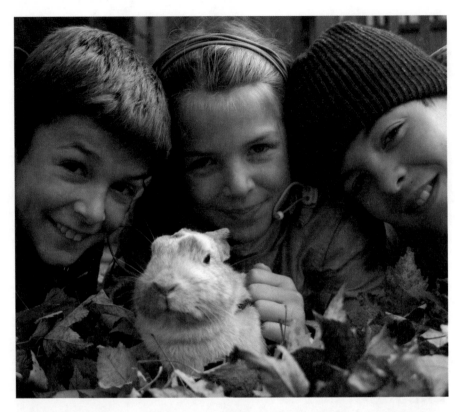

A better quality of life will benefit the whole family. As you enter your life swap, it is an ideal opportunity to make changes to family life. Spend more time with the children. Help the children to spend more time playing with friends or each other and less time watching TV or playing on computers.

This change is for the whole family. All family members should be involved. It must be fun and exciting for everyone. Children can help in the garden; have their own vegetable patch, keep hens or have other animals as pets. They can also participate in the community and get involved with village activities.

Children are very adaptable and there are benefits to be found in smaller schools; healthier living, more time spent outdoors, a more social environment, better food and generally the opportunity to live life at a slower more relaxed pace. They may need encouraging and coaxing into accepting the new way of life, but once they start enjoying it there will be no stopping them.

Personal development

Taking control of your life is hugely empowering. It has something to do with walking away from the 'pack', being your own person, deciding not to conform, being a maverick or being more self-sufficient. Any sort of change or life swap will ensure that you learn new skills. By living a different life, you are experiencing new things. It will be a mind-expanding experience. For those people who venture into buying or running their own business, the change is enormous and the skills and knowledge accrued during this undertaking will be vast.

The risks involved with swapping your life are huge in themselves, but making a success of it will give you tremendous confidence in your own ability. It will not all be easy and plain sailing, there will be hurdles to jump and doubts to overcome. Every now and again, you may even look back and think, 'What have I done?' Remember you have reached out, grasped life and made the most out of every day. People who downshift are proud of their achievement of trying something different and experiencing new things that others will never discover.

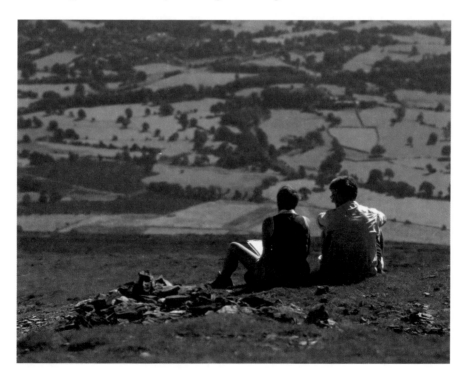

A richer life

Your life swap can offer you a much more complete existence. Your life will become multi-faceted. Your old life was dominated by work, getting the kids to school, housework, and then more work. There wasn't time for hobbies, community life or sport. Now you should have more time for lots of things. Getting out of the fast lane is liberating. You may find yourself just as busy, but you will be able to do a greater variety of things and they will be the things you choose to do.

Downshifting is almost a misnomer. Downshifting sounds as though it is a compacting and restricting experience. It is, in fact, the exact opposite. During your life swap you will expand. You will find yourself doing things you never thought you would do, achieving things you never thought you could achieve. You will be stepping off into the unknown.

The journey of living through a life swap is enriching and one of immense personal growth. It is the 21st century equivalent of being an 18th century explorer. You will learn so much more about the undiscovered you!

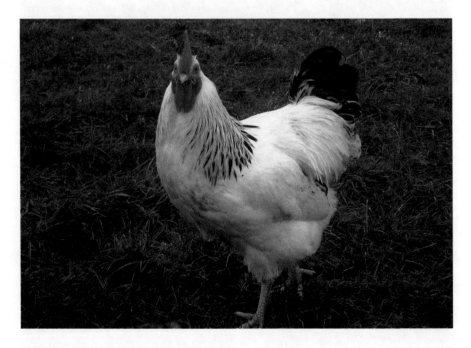

8

Ten top tips for a successful life swap

We have now covered many of the issues that confront us when thinking about making a life swap. If you follow the steps in this book and spend some time understanding the dream versus the reality, then you will have a good idea of whether a life swap is for you.

If you are still unsure here are **ten top tips** that summarise the issues raised in the previous chapters.

1 Never make a change in your life unless you know why you are doing it

The first thing to do if you are thinking about starting a new life is to find out what it is in your present life that is making you dissatisfied. It is really important to sort out where you are now before you make the leap to somewhere else.

2 Never make a change in your life unless you know where you are going

Find out, in your own mind, what sort of life you want to lead before you make any big decisions or plans.

Make sure you know what you want your life to look and feel like eventually.

3 You don't have to make a huge leap to improve your quality of life

Look at what is making you unhappy. Do you need a completely new start or do you just need to start living your life differently? Would more leisure time satisfy your need for change? Would your life improve by working smarter and improving your time management?

Sort out your finances

4

Spend some time sorting out how much money you need to live on, taking into consideration how much it costs you to live and work where you are now. Remember it costs money to go to work – travel, work clothes, equipment, bought lunches etc.

Try and work out how long you could survive without a full-time income (see page 85 for the cashflow spreadsheet).

If you want to make a new start, how much money will you need to have?

Remember, mortgages can be difficult to get if you have been self-employed for less than three years.

Give yourself some breathing space

5

If your finances will allow it, try to give yourself some breathing space between leaving your old life and starting you new life. Give yourself time to think and plan.

You also need time to physically and mentally adjust to your new life.

If you are going to make a life change – it must be for the better

6

Make sure that anything you plan to do in the future is going to help you achieve a better quality of life than you have now. A life with more time to do the things you want; those things that will make you feel fulfilled.

Do something you really enjoy or that gives you more control over your life.

7 Do not turn your back on all the skills you have acquired in your present life

Utilise the skills you already have.

If you need new skills try and learn them before you start your new life. This could be anything from cabinet making, horticulture and building, to keeping chickens.

8 Surround yourself with friends and family who support your move

Try and spend time with those around you who are as excited about your new life as you are, who admire your courage and will support you through the move.

You may have friends and family who will try to put you off changing your life – mostly for their own reasons.

Try to distance yourself from them as they will put doubts in your mind and may cause you to compromise on some really important issues. If you really want to paint and open your own gallery, don't let people talk you into starting off small, painting at home in your spare time and putting some pictures in local galleries to test the market. This might seem good advice, but if creating your own space is going to be your inspiration to paint, their limiting idea just won't work for you.

9 Stop spending

A life change or downshift will cost money and will generally mean that you have a reduced income.

Try to stop spending and be much more thoughtful about what you buy and what you really need.

Think about your list of 'wants' and try and change it to a list of 'needs'. You may be surprised at the outcome because many of the things you thought you wanted, you don't need.

GET HELP AND ADVICE

10

Do not try to change your life or start a new life without seeking help and advice. For every happy tale of downshifting, there is an even sorrier tale of those that didn't make it.

• Talk to other people who have downshifted

• Read books on life change and downshifting

• Talk to professionals like solicitors, accountants, financial advisors, banks etc

• Talk to other people who have changed their own life or downshifted, who can help you make sure you are making the right decisions for you and your family

• Talk to an expert in managing life change such as those at Stepping Off who will have with an objective view of your plans. They will help you clarify your options, help you make better decisions and plan a future that is right for you – visit www.steppingoff.co.uk

If you think that a life swap is for you, then the success will be in the planning. Take time to get the plans right. This is not a short-term goal.

You might plan your new life for 12 months or more. First, you have to make the decision that you want to swap your life. Then you will be able to look into your future options. When you have decided on the best option for you and your family, you will have lots of things to do and to decide on.

• What gear are you going to downshift to

• If you move, what geographical areas do you like

• Locations, houses and schools

• Give in and work your notice

• Find new work, business or premises

• Acquire new skills

• Sort out your finances and lots more . . .

Goal setting

Try to look at the whole issue as a big project and manage each stage. Work out what has to be done, break it down into small steps and set yourself realistic timescales within which to achieve them. This whole project could be a six-month or a five-year goal, but within that you will have other short and medium-term goals.

Remember, the most important thing about goal setting is to make sure that your goals are achievable and every time you reach and achieve one of your goals make sure that you reward yourself.

Your new life

So what is it going to feel like as you wake up on the first morning of your new life?

You can expect to feel tired, excited, terrified and exhilarated all at the same time. Try and hang on to the excitement. Change can be stressful and there will be lots to do, especially if you have moved house. Don't let it get you down. This is a fantastic thing you are doing. It is a great opportunity to live your life differently. Keep that thought always at the front of your mind.

The ultimate purpose of a life swap is to move towards a better life. Take time to get things right. This will not happen overnight. You and your family will need time to adjust and settle in. You will go through all sorts of emotions, doubts and panics over the following months, but it is all part of living through change and you will come to terms with them in time.

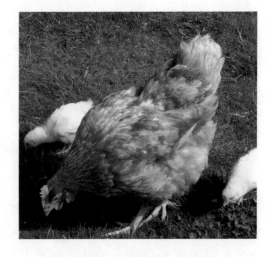

Advice from others who have swapped their lives

- Be prepared for anything!

- Make sure your relationship is strong enough to cope with the changes, stresses and strains

- Do not live in the house you are renovating...buy a luxury caravan and stay in it until all the mess is cleared, then sell the caravan!

- Only take on what you think you can do

- Finances – be realistic about what money you need. Don't do it until you have enough

- Give yourselves a break and a pat on the back now and then

- Stop and take stock of your achievements

- Make sure you adjust your mind to your new life

- Have fun and make it enjoyable

- Allow some time for you and your family. Whatever sort of work you go into, try and give your mind and body a break before you launch yourself into your new life.

The creepies!

'The creepies' are what we call those dark thoughts, doubts and panics that develop as you embark on your life swap! For most people, downshifting is a huge leap and as they give up jobs, sell homes and move, there is a real feeling of burning bridges. The security has gone. What happens if we have made a mistake? What happens if it all goes wrong? What happens if we don't make any money?

Try and put these thoughts to one side and look at what you are doing practically. Keep on top of your targets and goals and work hard to maintain your timescales.

Leaving is as difficult as starting again. There may be a genuine sense of loss, which can trigger emotions that are akin to mourning. Don't be surprised if at times you feel sad, you have every right to, but try to counter these feelings by getting excited about what you are doing in your new life and what you are achieving.

More than anything, you will worry about your finances and money. Strange things can happen – some people ignore the fact that they have very little income and keep spending! Not advisable. Others just stop spending. They put themselves through some sort of self-imposed insolvency; they never use the phone, only shop at cut-price stores, and never go out! This is actually good; it focuses the mind very firmly on your 'wants' and 'needs'. These feelings will become less extreme with time.

Every time something doesn't go to plan the 'creepies' will return. It may be an up-hill struggle to find definition in your new life. Many of us define ourselves by what we do. If you have just given up your job and are doing nothing or are about to start something completely new, then you may well be in some sort of turmoil as to your identity. This will be short-lived and if anticipated can be minimised.

Making new friends may be challenging to some people and it is not always easy fitting into a new community. Not all communities welcome newcomers with open arms. Finding a new social circle can take time, so if it is important to you persevere. It only takes one contact or one invitation to set the ball rolling.

Don't look back!

We have already mentioned the emotions you may experience when you hear about the successes of past friends and colleagues. Don't let them unsettle you. They may be exaggerated anyway because they are jealous of you. Look at all you have achieved, know that your quality of life is good and that you are living the life you want to.

Be satisfied with what you have and what you have achieved. Look around you and you will see that what you have experienced in your life is already more than most other people could ever hope to achieve.

Be satisfied, knowing that you have sculpted the life you are living. It hasn't been thrown together through a series of coincidences or happenings or been moulded by other people. You made definite decisions to put yourself in the place you are now.

There may be occasions when you think back to the days when money was plentiful, but it is important to recognise how much better your life is now and how much happier you are. You will have things that money just couldn't buy you in your old life, like time, control, space and fulfillment.

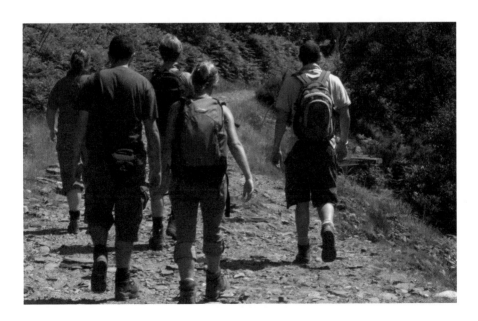

Look forward!

Enjoy, enjoy, enjoy! Take pride in what you have done. It is easy to conform and live like everyone else, the difficult bit is to step out on your own and define your life in unconventional terms. Be proud of your courage.

Your life is stretching out in front of you, the world is at your feet and there is nothing that you cannot do if you put your mind to it. If things go wrong and mistakes are made – well at least you gave it a go. At least you tried, and in trying you will have gained valuable life experience. Do not regret anything that goes wrong; move on to do different and varied things.

When you are 85 years old and looking back on your life, don't worry about any 'what ifs' because life is full of imponderables. Don't allow yourself any 'if onlys,' they are regrets and life is just too short to have regrets.

Go out there and live, make the most of every day and revel in your life swap.

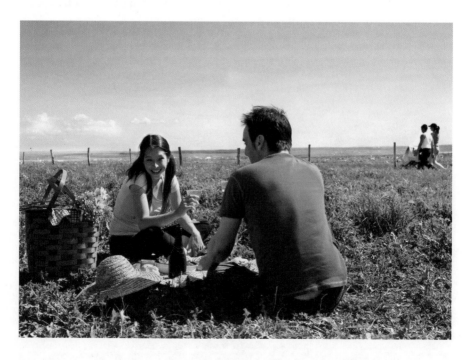

9

Case studies

Finding the right gear to live in isn't easy and not everyone gets it right first time. There are a number of people who move down a gear and then, a few years later, when they feel they are ready for the next step, they move down further gears.

Some people cross-shift into a busier life than they had before, but this time they enjoy different successes. Maybe they are living in the country or running their own business, but either way they are enjoying a better quality of life.

Some people downshift a gear too far and never really settle in that gear. After a while they move back up a gear or two, but keep hold of many of the lessons learnt from their life swap.

Sadly, for some the experience of a life swap is not a happy one. This can be for a number of reasons, but mostly this will be due to a lack of planning and research or not spending sufficient time working out who they are, where they are and where they want to be before they make the move.

Here are a few examples of families and individuals who have recently swapped their lives.

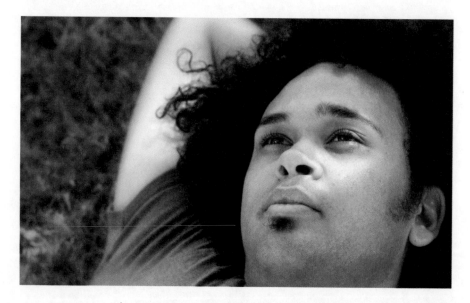

Wendy and Simon

When Wendy and Simon met, Simon was a journalist for an evening news-paper with a background in international hotel management and working in five star hotels all over the world. Wendy was in human resources.

They took the first step towards a life swap when they bought a share of a restaurant in Mayfair. Simon put his writing career on the back burner and ran the restaurant full-time, while Wendy continued to work in recruitment.

They became ever more disillusioned with London life, with the traffic, rush, noise and pace of everyday life. When they saw an old castle advertised for sale, on a whim, they went to have a look. Neither of them believed they were going to look at their future, but they hadn't even reached the end of the drive before they knew they could make the castle their home. And so they made a life swap and embarked on a project to breathe life into the once grand old house and open it up as a guest house.

"We can honestly say that moving from our jobs and lives in London was one of the best decisions we have ever made. That's not to say the transition - or our lives here - have been easy! The work has been hard, at times seemingly impossible. But every achievement has been so satisfying."

Since then, they have created new suites, renovated a cottage, and landscaped the grounds. They are licensed for civil marriages, have won Les Routiers Bed and Breakfast of the year, have achieved five red diamonds from the AA and appeared in the Good Hotel Guide.

It has been a labour of love and extremely hard work. Several years on, they have a thriving business, they employ a number of staff and they are able to create more time for themselves and their family.

Simon and Wendy have cross-shifted - swapping one busy life for another. Simon objects to people who talk about their move as downshifting. He sees his life as having expanded, not downsized. He explains that even though they left the city to move to the country, he now has much more than he used to have. They have increased their income, they have a better standard of living, own more property and are much more successful than they were in their old life. They are much happier and state that despite all the hard work; they now have control over their life. They have time to do more things, their quality of life has improved and they wouldn't go back for anything.

Graham and Sarah

Graham had a very good job and a high salary. Sarah was working her way up the ladder in London, but spent much of her time commuting. They juggled childcare between themselves and the childminders. Graham had become disillusioned with his organisation, how he was treated and the support he received. He decided that he wanted out and they looked to swap their lives. They decided that they would give it all up, move to France, buy a tumble down property and do it up.

This they did. Graham had some limited DIY experience, but a lot of enthusiasm and Sarah had always wanted to live in France. Once they were settled and the work was underway, Sarah was asked to do some part-time work for one of her old companies. To supplement the income, she agreed. This work was extended and she was soon working harder and was in demand from other international clients. She spent much of her time commuting to the UK!

They loved their rural life in France, growing vegetables and keeping chickens. But, eventually, they decided that as Sarah was becoming more and more in demand, in order for her to fulfill her potential, they would move back to the UK.

They did not, however, turn their backs on all that had appealed to them, and all that they had learnt about rural living. Once back, they found another restoration 'project' for Graham and they set about re-building their lives, whilst still living more simply. They are now living a very 'green' existence. Graham is enjoying his new challenge and Sarah works as a consultant. She has more control over her working hours and her time. She manages to work from home most of the time. Sarah has moved back up a gear, but is still living a couple of gears down from where she started.

Although their downshifting to France did not last, they are happy because they are still living a simpler, rural life, here in the UK.

Inger

Inger downshifted from the Southeast to Devon, and then she did it all over again.

Inger was well-paid and far too busy. She was cash rich, but time poor. She had had enough of the fast pace life and dreamed of living in a remote area and working on a conservation or environmental project.

Although she had extensive management experience, she knew that she had little relevant experience in conservation. To improve and broaden her skills base she left her job and through some very careful financial planning was able to visit New Zealand where she worked as a volunteer for a number of months on three different conservation projects. This was a superb experience.

On her return, she discovered that finding a job was hard and her financial situation was stressful. After about three months, she found a job in the southwest. Her cut in salary was hard to come to terms with, but she managed to adjust her spending to her new income and life settled down. She was happy living in the country, but her dream was still to be living in a really remote area and working in a more hands-on way in conservation.

Out of the blue, she was offered her perfect job in New Zealand. She gave up her newly found life in Devon in order to start all over again in a remote part of the country, some two hours drive from the nearest supermarket! She is now living only a few minutes walk from where she works and really feels that her job is in an area that fits her interests.

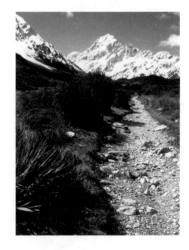

Inger moved down through the gears twice and is now very happy living her dream. Inger stepped off and was successful because she did not try and achieve her long-term goals straight away. She was careful, thought about what she really wanted from life and then, through a programme of work experience and gradual change, she ended up living the life she had always dreamed of in New Zealand.

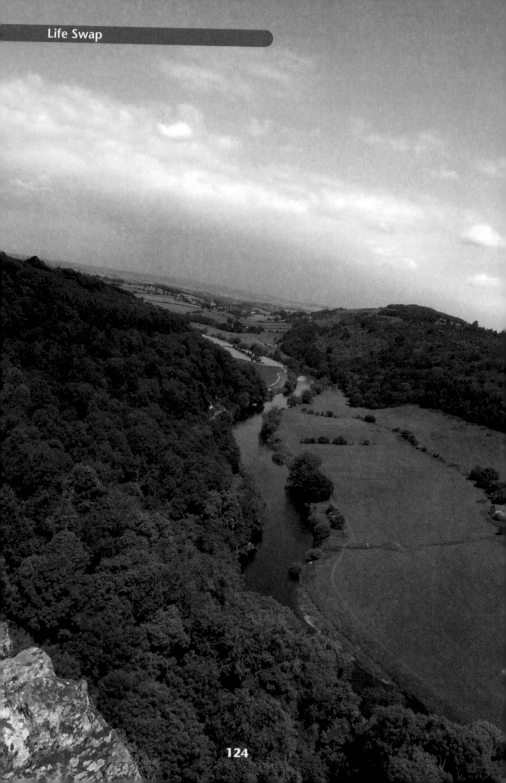

Robert and Ruth

Robert and Ruth led a comfortable life in the Southeast. They lived outside London and had a high standard of living. Robert was successful and Ruth enjoyed her life, being involved in the community and voluntary work.

However they had a romantic idea of living in the countryside, so they decided that they would move to a more rural location and start their own business. Robert gave up his job; they sold their house and rented an unusual folly in a village. They put some of their money from their house into setting up their own business.

Four years on, and the business is ticking over, but not thriving. Robert has taken a part-time job back in the Southeast and is away from home a lot. Ruth is finding the business difficult and really misses her previous standard of life.

Money is a big thing for them. They enjoyed having money and all the things that money can buy and are finding that a simpler and better quality of life does not make up for the loss of income.

Sadly, the business is not worth sufficient to allow them to sell and move back down to the Southeast where house prices have risen. Robert could get a full-time job, but they have little capital, so again they would be looking at modest accommodation if they moved and Ruth has had enough of modest living. The best they can hope for is that their business improves greatly and they become more successful or that Robert can get a full-time job nearer home. Ruth has thought about wrapping up the business and getting a full-time job herself, but sees little that appeals to her.

This is a sad story, but is not uncommon. Ruth and Robert had a dream, but they did not spend enough time analysing what they really wanted from a life swap and why they wanted to move. With hindsight, they acknowledge that neither of them were unhappy with their lives, they just had a romantic dream about replicating their existence in a different location. In addition, Robert turned his back on his skills base and then found that between them they did not possess all the required skills necessary to make a success of the business they had started up. This meant that in order to survive, they had to buy in those skills, which reduced their profits dramatically.

Helen and Jane

Helen and Jane had already swapped their working lives and started up their own successful business looking after people's pets. Although their life had improved, the environment around them remained the same. They lived in an inner city area that was inhospitable and aggressive. They were still faced with road rage, cultural hatred, wanton damage and mindless abuse.

They decided that they wanted to get away and lead a simpler life. The thought of renovating a house and starting a guesthouse seemed like a good idea - only they decided on a property in France. Finding the right premises and moving took nearly two years and that was before they had even started the renovation!

Their B&B is now up and running, doing well in season and they are confident it will improve, as they get known. But, the drop in income has been difficult for them and Jane has occasionally come back to the UK, on short term contracts, to improve their cash flow. This flexibility and adaptability is essential when making a life swap, particularly in the early days when times can be hard. Both Helen and Jane have worked hard to set up this business and although the financial situation has sometimes meant they have had to take on work back in the UK, they still feel that their standard and quality of life has improved and they wouldn't change the lives they have now for anything.

The best part of their new life according to Helen is that they are in control.

> " It's up to us how we go about things, the standard to which we do them, how we organise our time and when we take holidays. Where we live is so tranquil, the air is clean and there is no noise pollution - it is really quiet. And we don't even have TV. We have never been happier".

Could this be you?

Stepping Off – the course

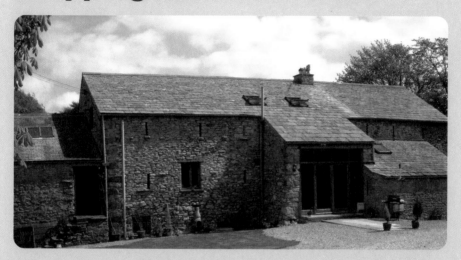

The mission of Stepping Off is to help those wanting to escape the rat race and to make sure that they do not leap from the frying pan into the fire. There are complex motivators that steer people towards any major life change, and we have developed some simple tools to establish what their real priorities are during this process.

We offer relaxing day and weekend courses in a beautiful converted Westmorland barn where people can come and escape the pressures of everyday living and sort out their future. We specialise in helping people work out what they really want out of life, where they want to be and how to get there. We help with every aspect of changing your life, from simple time management to complete downshifting. We even help people work through what stops them doing and being what they really want.

Clients of Stepping Off enjoy time in a wonderful country house environment where the focus is on the individual and their future. They also enjoy great local food, have time out to walk on the fells or relax in front of a log fire and will come away revitalized with an action plan on how to achieve their new life.

www.steppingoff.co.uk

The reality of life change

The company motto at Stepping Off is - **"You hold on to your dream, while we help you live through the reality."**

Jo and Georgina certainly know about the dream and the reality. Escaping the rat race doesn't always come easy when you have had a rewarding and successful career. When they wanted to downshift themselves, they found that there was a real lack of specific advice available to help them achieve their ambitions. Consequently, they made some mistakes and there are a lot of things they could have done differently to make the transition easier.

As Jo reflects, "Embarking on this sort of life change is momentous, yet people do it without really thinking it through. For every happy story of people success-fully downshifting there is a sorrier tale of those who get it wrong. We were lucky. It makes sense to give yourself the best chance and learn a few useful hints from those who have successfully achieved what you are trying to do".

Downshifting is, one way or another, becoming more and more fashionable – as much on TV as in reality! How many people do you know that have been saying for years "One of these days I'll leave" "I wish I could give it all up" "I'm hoping for redundancy" "I always wanted to be..." "Next year I won't work so hard."

The ethos of Stepping Off - and one that they are really enthusiastic about is that there really is no time like the present to begin to enjoy life. What better way to start a new chapter in your life than with a relaxing weekend away where the focus is completely on you, and what you want to do, with people there to help you get it right!

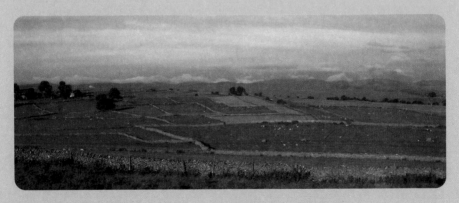